A Physician's Guide to the Management of Huntington's Disease

Third Edition

Martha Nance, M.D.
Director, HDSA Center of Excellence at Hennepin County Medical Center
Medical Director, Struthers Parkinson's Center, Minneapolis, MN
Adjunct Professor, Department of Neurology, University of Minnesota

Jane S. Paulsen, Ph.D.
Director HDSA Center of Excellence at the University of Iowa
Professor of Neurology, Psychiatry, Psychology, and Neuroscience,
University of Iowa Carver College of Medicine, Iowa City, IA
Principal Investigator, PREDICT-HD, Study of Early Markers in HD

Adam Rosenblatt, M.D.
Director, HDSA Center of Excellence at Johns Hopkins, Baltimore Maryland
Associate Professor of Psychiatry, and Director of Neuropsychiatry,
Johns Hopkins University School of Medicine

Vicki Wheelock, M.D.
Director, HDSA Center of Excellence at University of California
Clinical Professor, Neurology, University of California,
Davis Medical Center, Sacramento, CA
Site Investigator, Huntington Study Group

Editors: Debra Lovecky
Director of Programs, Services & Advocacy, HDSA

Karen Tarapata

Designer: J&R Graphics

Printed with funding from an unrestricted educational grant provided by Lundbeck

1

Disclaimer

The indications and dosages of drugs in this book have either been recommended in the medical literature or conform to the practices of physicians' expert in the care of people with Huntington's Disease. The medications do not necessarily have specific approval from the Food and Drug Administration for the indications and dosages for which they are recommended in this guide. The package insert for each drug should be consulted for uses and dosage approved by the FDA. Because standards for dosage change, it is advisable to keep abreast of revised recommendations, particularly those concerning new drugs.

Statements and opinions expressed in this book are not necessarily those of the Huntington's Disease Society of America, Inc., nor does HDSA promote, endorse, or recommend any treatment or therapy mentioned herein. The lay reader should consult a physician or other appropriate health care professional regarding any advice, treatment or therapy set forth in this book.

No part of *A Physician's Guide to the Management of Huntington's Disease* (Third Edition) may be reproduced in any way without the express written permission of the Huntington's Disease Society of America.

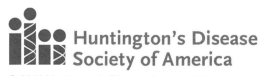

Huntington's Disease
Society of America

© 2011 Huntington's Disease Society of America
All rights reserved.
Printed in the United States of America

ISBN 978-1-4507-7064-4

9 781450 770644

Table of Contents

Preface

It has been more than ten years since the last edition of *A Physician's Guide to the Management of Huntington's Disease*. In that time, a great deal has been learned about HD. We now have a much better understanding of its genetic, biochemical, and neuroanatomic basis.

We also know more than ever about the earliest stages of HD. Since the last edition, long term observational studies, such as PREDICT-HD, have provided new insights into the prodrome of the disease. As an example, research indicates that changes in cognition and executive functioning are detectable as much as 8-15 years before the motor symptoms emerge. How this information is to be used in a clinical setting is still under discussion, but it may allow people with HD to exert more control over their future, make informed choices, and establish support systems in advance of need.

As in previous editions, the guide is principally organized into three areas around the movement, cognitive and psychiatric disorders associated with HD, and several generally accepted pharmacological and non-pharmacological treatments are presented for each problem, where possible. This edition also covers new topics of interest to the physician, including multidisciplinary team care for HD, Juvenile onset HD, management of late stage HD and the prodrome of HD. Finally, there is a review of current trends in HD research.

While there have been many breakthroughs in our understanding of HD, research has not, as yet, delivered a treatment that can slow, halt or reverse the progression of HD. One medication for the symptomatic treatment of chorea has received FDA approval, and other promising therapeutic compounds and drugs are currently in clinical trials. Other drugs, already FDA approved for other conditions, are also undergoing clinical trials to see if they may be effective in treating HD.

In the absence of a cure for the disease, people with HD, their families, and their physicians must find creative means to meet the goals of treatment for HD, which are to reduce the burden of symptoms, maximize function and optimize quality of life.

We remain dedicated to the belief that while HD is currently incurable, there is always something that can be done to help the person with HD. This guide is designed to help doctors understand the complexities of HD and the possibilities for thoughtful and creative treatment of its symptoms.

Chapter 1

Overview and Principles of Treatment

Adam Rosenblatt, M.D.

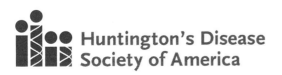
**Huntington's Disease
Society of America**

Overview

Huntington's Disease (HD) is a hereditary neurodegenerative disorder caused by an expansion of a repeating CAG triplet series in the huntingtin gene on chromosome 4, which results in a protein with an abnormally long polyglutamine sequence. HD is one of a larger family of polyglutamine repeat disorders, all of which are neurodegenerative diseases. It is inherited in an autosomal dominant fashion, so that each child of an affected parent has a 50% chance of developing the disease. There is currently no cure or treatment which can halt, slow or reverse the progression of the disease.

The HD gene was identified in 1993. It contains a repeating sequence of three base-pairs, called a "triplet repeat" or "trinucleotide repeat." An excess number of CAG repeats in the gene results in a protein containing an excess number of glutamine units. The normal function of huntingtin is not known, but the expanded polyglutamine sequence in the huntingtin protein is in some way toxic to brain cells. Just as in other polyglutamine expansion disorders, certain neurons appear to be more vulnerable to damage in HD. Atrophy is most marked in the corpus striatum of the basal ganglia, including the caudate and putamen. In later phases of the disease, other regions of the brain are also affected.

The Progression of HD

Huntington's Disease manifests as a triad of motor, cognitive, and psychiatric symptoms which begin insidiously and progress over many years, until the death of the individual. The average length of survival after clinical diagnosis is typically 10-20 years, but some people have lived thirty or forty years. Late stage HD may last up to a decade or more.

Prodrome

The clinical diagnosis of HD is traditionally based on the observation of involuntary (choreiform) movements in a person with an appropriate family history, and supportive social history (such as a decline in function or insidious onset of mood disturbance).

In the last decade, observational studies on the earliest stages of HD have revealed that there is a prodrome of HD (symptoms indicating the presence of a disease process prior to the development of the full clinical syndrome) that may appear up to 15 years before the onset of motor symptoms. Prodromal cognitive changes have been observed in about 40% of individuals studied and are detectable in more than 70% of those close to a diagnosis of manifest HD. Several studies have suggested that cognitive and behavioral impairments are greater sources of impaired functioning than the movement disorder in persons with HD, both in the work place and at home.

The Disorders of HD

The *movement disorder* of HD includes emergence of involuntary movements (chorea) and the impairment of voluntary movements, which result in reduced manual dexterity, slurred speech, swallowing difficulties, problems with balance, and falls. Chorea typically progresses through the middle stages of HD, but often declines as rigidity increases in the later stages.

The *cognitive disorder* of HD is characterized by a reduction of speed and flexibility in mental processing. Cognitive losses accumulate and people with HD develop more global impairments in the later stages of the disease. Memory, language, and conceptual ability persist, but limited output impedes our ability to assess them.

The *psychiatric disorder* in HD is less predictable. People with HD may suffer from depression and other conditions found in the general population, such as mania, obsessive compulsive disorder, or various forms of psychosis. However, almost all people with HD will manifest disease-specific personality and behavioral changes as part of what might be termed a hypofrontal or dysexecutive syndrome, characterized by apathy, irritability, impulsivity, and obsessionality, with potentially severe consequences for the HD person's marital, social, and economic well-being.

The disorders of HD cannot be considered in isolation. Disabilities in one area will lead to problems in another. For example, treatments for the psychiatric disorder may have a negative impact on the movement disorder. Changes in cognition have an effect on the ability to perform physical tasks such as driving or cooking. Few other diseases have this level of interconnected disabilities, affecting all areas of an individual's life.

Age of Onset

People with HD show a wide range in the age of onset. While most people with HD develop the motor symptoms in their forties and fifties, subtle changes may arise much earlier. Knowledge of the typical age of onset sometimes leads physicians to miss the diagnosis, mistakenly believing the person to be too old or too young to develop HD. About 10% have onset of motor symptoms after age 60 and 10% have Juvenile onset HD, where symptoms manifest before age 20.

Stages of HD

HD can be roughly divided into three phases (although a five-stage scale is sometimes used). In *early stage* HD, individuals are largely functional and may continue to work, drive, handle money, and live independently. Symptoms may include minor involuntary movements, subtle loss of coordination, difficulty thinking through complex problems, and perhaps some depression, irritability, or disinhibition.

In *middle stage* HD, individuals lose the ability to work or drive and may no longer be able to manage their own finances or perform their own household chores, but will be able to eat, dress, and attend to personal hygiene with assistance. Chorea may be prominent, and people with HD have increasing difficulty with voluntary motor tasks. There may be problems with swallowing, balance, falls, and weight loss. Problem solving becomes more difficult because individuals cannot sequence, organize, or prioritize information.

In *late stage* HD, individuals require assistance in all activities of daily living. Although they are often nonverbal and bedridden in the end stages, it is important to note that people with HD seem to retain some comprehension. Chorea may be severe, but more often it is replaced by rigidity, dystonia, and bradykinesia. Psychiatric symptoms may occur at any point in the course of the disease, but are harder to recognize and treat late in the disease because of communication difficulties.

Several schemes for staging HD exist. One of the most commonly used is a rating scale based on functional abilities, the Total Functional Capacity Rating Scale (see page 8). This scale rates the person's level of independence in five domains:

occupation, ability to manage finances, ability to perform domestic chores, ability to perform personal activities of daily living, and setting for level of care. Some clinicians use the TFC score to determine the disease stage according to the Shoulson and Fahn rating scale.

Total Functional Capacity Rating Scale[1] (Source: UHDRS[2])		
Domain	**Ability**	**Score**
Occupation	Unable	0
	Marginal work only	1
	Reduced capacity for usual job	2
	Normal	3
Finances	Unable	0
	Major assistance	1
	Slight assistance	2
	Normal	3
Domestic Chores	Unable	0
	Impaired	1
	Normal	2
Activities of Daily Living	Total care	0
	Gross tasks only	1
	Minimal impairment	2
	Normal	3
Care level	Full-time nursing care	0
	Home for chronic care	1
	Home	2
TOTAL	Range 0 - 13	

Shoulson and Fahn Staging Scale[1]

TFC Total Score	**Stage**
11 - 13	I
7 - 10	II
3 - 6	III
1 - 2	IV
0	V

1 Shoulson I, Kurlan R, Rubin AJ et al. Assessment of functional capacity in neurodegenerative movement disorders: Huntington's disease as a prototype, in Munsat TL (ed): Quantification of Neurological Deficit. Boston: Butterworth, 1989, pp 271-283.

2 The Huntington Study Group. Unified Huntington's Disease Rating Scale: reliability and consistency. Mov Disord 1996; 11:136-142.

Table 1.

Progression of symptoms and disability in a typical person with Huntington's Disease

Cognitive symptoms (dementia)

Motor symptoms
Impaired volitional movements
Chorea
Dystonia

Psychiatric/behavioral symptoms

Weight loss

Life milestones
- Parent diagnosed with HD; Suicide gesture
- Marriage
- First child born
- Suicide attempt
- Disabled from work; affected parent dies
- Placed in long-term care facility

Disease milestones
- First awareness of risk of HD
- Positive predictive gene test
- Diagnosis
- Death

Total Functional Capacity (0-13 points)

Stage 1: 11-13 points; changes in work, role within family

Stage 2: 7-10 points; issues include work, finances, driving; able to live at home with minimal supervision

Stage 3: 3-6 points; impaired ADLs (activities of daily living), needs supervision

Stage 4: 1-2 points; needs assistance with most ADLs, 24-hour care appropriate

Stage 5: 0 points; needs assistance with all ADLs; progression to terminal stages

Y-axis values: 14, 12, 10, 8, 6, 4, 2, 0

Age (Years)

X-axis values: 0, 5, 10, 15, 20, 25, 30, 35, 40, 45, 50

Table 1 shows the interrelated symptoms of HD along the typical continuum of the disease. Some symptoms will fluctuate in severity during the progression of the disease, others will steadily worsen.

It is important to remember that each person with HD is different and while the disease has an overall progression, the onset of symptoms and their severity is unique to each case.

Juvenile onset HD

HD with onset in childhood has somewhat different features. Chorea is a much less prominent feature, and may be absent altogether. Initial symptoms usually include attentional deficits, behavioral disorders, school failure, dystonia, bradykinesia, and sometimes tremor. Seizures, rarely found in adults, may occur in this juvenile form. Juvenile onset HD tends to follow a more rapid course, with survival less than 15 years.

Diagnosis and Genetic Testing

The clinical diagnosis of HD is typically made on the basis of family history and the presence of an otherwise unexplained characteristic movement disorder, and may be confirmed by a gene test. The gene test is particularly useful when there is an unknown, or negative family history (as occurs in cases of early parental death, adoption, misdiagnosis, or non-paternity) or when the family history is positive, but the symptoms are atypical.

It is important to remember that the gene test only determines whether or not the HD-causing genetic expansion is present, and not whether an individual's current symptoms are caused by the HD gene. This is particularly relevant in cases of possible Juvenile onset HD in which a child at-risk for HD may have non-specific academic or behavioral problems.

The diagnosis of HD remains a clinical diagnosis. The motor disorder can be delineated and followed longitudinally using a quantitative examination designed for HD, such as the motor section of the Unified Huntington's Disease Rating Scale, which also includes a useful scale for functional capacity, or the Quantified Neurological Examination. Short cognitive tests such as the Mini-Mental State Examination are useful in following the cognitive disorder longitudinally, but lack sensitivity in certain areas which are affected in Huntington's Disease. A more sophisticated cognitive battery offers greater precision about the cognitive profile of HD.

The implications of the diagnosis of HD for the individual and family are profound, and provision should be made for genetic counseling of individuals before and after the testing process. Genetic counseling and genetic testing are discussed more fully in Chapter 2.

Guidelines for genetic testing are constantly under review and revision. It is recommended that physicians contact a genetic counselor at an HDSA Center of Excellence or visit the website of the Huntington's Disease Society of America, www.hdsa.org, to receive information on current best practices and the location of participating genetic testing centers.

Principles of Treatment

Caring for people with HD is both challenging and rewarding. At times, the lack of definitive treatments can be frustrating, but careful attention to the changing symptoms and good communication between professionals, family members, and affected individuals can contribute to the successful management of the disease. Because there are no treatments which can slow, halt, or reverse the course of the disease, the goals of treatment are to reduce the burden of symptoms, maximize function, and optimize quality of life.

Symptoms of HD evolve over time as a person passes through different stages of the disease. Symptoms also vary from individual to individual, even within a family. For example, one person may develop a severe mood disorder, requiring multiple hospitalizations, but have little motor disability at the time. The individual's brother may have debilitating motor symptoms at the same disease duration, but no mood disturbance at all. Thus interventions need to be tailored to individual symptoms, and fearful HD persons should be reassured that their symptoms may not necessarily resemble those of their relatives.

Treatment information and functional scales presented in this guide represent the best efforts of the authors to provide physicians and neurologists with recommendations and tools that are based on published guidelines and reviews, tempered by the authors' professional and clinical experience. These treatment guidelines and assessment tools are constantly being improved and refined. It is recommended that the physician periodically visit the website of the Huntington Disease Society of America for information on the current best practices or consult with one of HDSA's 21 Centers of Excellence. A listing can be found on www.hdsa.org.

Medications

HD is a progressive disease. The symptoms evolve over time and medications which were effective in the early stages may be unnecessary or problematic in later stages, and vice versa. For example, medications that are started in the early to middle stages to control chorea may exacerbate the rigidity and bradykinesia of the later stages, and result in delirium or over-sedation. The medication list and the rationale for each medication should be re-evaluated at regular intervals. Sometimes the most helpful intervention a physician can perform is to discontinue an unnecessary drug.

People with HD, like others with diseases and injuries of the brain, are highly vulnerable to side effects, particularly cognitive side effects, of medications. The physician should begin with low doses and advance medicines slowly. Polypharmacy should be avoided where possible. Many of the drugs used in treating symptoms of HD, such as antidepressants, neuroleptics and tetrabenazine will not have immediate efficacy; people with HD need to be told that they may feel worse before they feel better, because they will experience the side effects before the beneficial effects have appeared.

Pharmacologic interventions should not be launched in isolation, but in a setting of education, social support, and environmental management. Symptomatic treatment of HD needs to be approached like any other medical problem. The clinician should elicit the details of the symptom, its character, onset and duration, and its context including precipitating, exacerbating and ameliorating factors. A differential diagnosis should be generated, non-pharmacologic interventions should be considered, and the clinician should have a way of determining whether the goals of treatment are being met and should formulate a contingency plan if treatment is not working. Sharing some of this reasoning process with the person with HD and their family can be reassuring.

Treatment Guidelines

Throughout this guide, we have provided guidelines for pharmacological treatments for the symptoms of HD. The suggested medications and dosages are those that are commonly used in the HDSA Centers of Excellence and represent the combined clinical experience of the authors.

Too often, HD families complain of under-treatment of symptoms by physicians and neurologists. While the disease is currently incurable, treatments exist that can substantially relieve symptoms and improve quality of life.

The physician who wishes to review treatment guidelines beyond those presented in this guide may reference the treatment guidelines created by the European Huntington's Disease Network (EHDN), the 2007 treatment review of Drs. Bonelli and Hofmann of studies for chorea and the psychiatric symptoms of HD that have been published in scientific journals since 1990, or the work of the Huntington's Disease DrugWorks. Information on these treatment guidelines may be found in Appendix II of this guide, Chapter Notes.

Caregivers as Informants

People with HD will often be accompanied by a caregiver on visits to the doctor. This caregiver can be a crucial informant, particularly in the later stages of the disease, when speech and cognitive difficulties may prevent a person with HD from supplying a history. However, both the person with HD and the caregiver may not feel comfortable discussing certain important issues in each other's presence, such as irritability, driving, relationship issues, or sexual problems. Therefore an effort should be made to speak to both individuals alone during the visit.

Benefits of Early Intervention

As stated earlier, the goals of treatment in HD are to reduce the burden of symptoms, maximize function and optimize quality of life. Allied health professionals have an important role to play in achieving these goals for the person with HD. Physicians are encouraged to use a team care model for treatment and refer the individual, as needed, to an occupational therapist, physical therapist, speech-language pathologist, and dietician/nutritionist who can help increase safety, functional independence and comfort in daily life.

Experimental and Alternative Treatments for HD

Physicians should help HD families distinguish between unproven remedies such as herbs, megadose vitamins, homeopathic preparations, or magnetic devices, and experimental treatments being researched in scientifically sound clinical studies.

A person with HD should be helped to understand that there is no substance, no matter how natural, which has pharmacologic activity without the potential for side effects, and that all treatments carry an element of risk. However, individuals should be encouraged to discuss therapies they are considering and not be afraid to tell their physicians that they are trying them. This will allow the doctor to help the person with HD to avoid dangerous or ineffective nostrums, and to monitor for side effects.

To minimize the risk for those who have chosen to pursue alternative therapies, the physician may offer the following principles: 1) Don't spend too much money, 2) Don't do something that common sense suggests is dangerous, and 3) Don't neglect or discontinue proven medical treatments which are having even a limited positive effect in favor of an unproven therapy making unfounded claims.

Physicians wishing to help a person with HD to locate clinical trials of experimental drugs and therapies should visit HDTrials.org; the HDSA website, www.hdsa.org; or the Huntington Study Group, www.huntington-study-group.org, which is an international consortium of scientific investigators from academic and research centers who are committed to cooperative planning, implementation, analysis and reporting of controlled clinical trials and other therapeutic research for HD.

Chapter 2

Genetic Counseling
and Genetic Testing

Martha Nance, M.D.

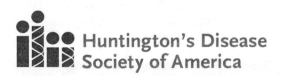 Huntington's Disease
Society of America

Genetic Counseling and Genetic Testing

A diagnosis of Huntington's Disease (HD) affects the entire extended family. The person who is diagnosed with HD grieves not only for himself, but also for his at-risk children, and a young adult child caring for an affected parent understands that the parent's disease could one day affect him.

The physician treating an HD family must be sensitive to the broad effect that the diagnosis will have on the family, and do his best to ensure that all family members have accurate information with which they can make informed decisions about genetic testing, reproduction, and financial and life planning. Even in the 21st century, almost 20 years after the HD gene was identified, misinformation and misunderstandings are common.

The Genetics of HD

HD is an autosomal dominant disease, which means it affects males and females with equal likelihood. Each child of an affected individual has the same 50% chance of inheriting the abnormal huntingtin gene, and therefore developing the disease one day. Inheriting a normal huntingtin gene from the unaffected parent does not prevent or counteract the disease-causing effects of the abnormal gene. In those rare cases where an individual carries two abnormal copies of the gene, the individual will develop HD, and each child has a 100% chance of inheriting an abnormal gene.

The Pattern of Inheritance in HD

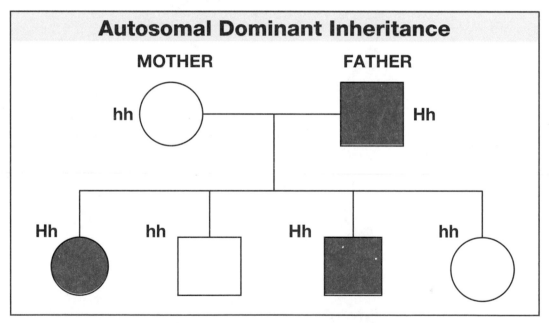

Understanding the huntingtin (IT-15) Gene and the huntingtin Protein

The huntingtin gene directs the cell to make huntingtin protein, whose functions within the cell are largely unknown. Huntingtin protein contains a sequence in which the amino acid glutamine is repeated a number of times. These glutamine residues are encoded in the gene by the DNA trinucleotide "CAG." The number of times that "CAG" is repeated (the CAG repeat number) determines the number of consecutive glutamines in that segment of the huntingtin protein. The huntingtin protein appears to be produced in equal quantities, whether it has a normal or excess number of glutamines, but the abnormally elongated protein appears to be processed aberrantly within the neurons, so that its fragments tend to accumulate over time into intranuclear inclusions. The details of this process and how it relates to the development of neurologic disease are still being studied.

Significance of CAG repeats in the huntingtin gene	
CAG repeat length	Interpretation
< 27	Normal
27-35	Normal, mutable (sometimes called the "intermediate range")
36-39	Abnormal, reduced penetrance (sometimes called the "indeterminate range")
≥ 40	Abnormal

The normal and abnormal CAG repeat number ranges have been determined by clinical experience which includes well over 10,000 affected individuals worldwide. Normal huntingtin genes contain 10-35 "CAG repeats." Individuals who have two copies of a normal huntingtin gene will not develop HD. Repeat sizes of 36 and above can be associated with the development of Huntington's Disease. CAG repeat numbers between 36 and 39 are associated with "reduced penetrance," meaning that not all carriers of these abnormal genes will develop diagnosable symptoms of HD within a normal lifespan. Individuals who have 40 or more CAG repeats in one of their huntingtin genes will develop HD if they live a normal lifespan.

Author's opinion:

A small number of unusual cases have been reported in the literature, including cases of apparent HD in people with <36 CAG repeats in their larger HD allele, and an individual who inherited an allele from an affected parent that contracted across the boundary (41 decreased to 35 CAG repeats). In addition, an occasional healthy person from a non-HD family, such as a spouse who has volunteered as a control, is found to have a CAG repeat in the "intermediate range" and becomes alarmed. Some of the cases include better documentation of clinical, genetic, or pathologic features than others. It is the author's opinion that the existence of these cases do not yet require us to change the established boundaries between "normal" and "abnormal" CAG repeat numbers. Any person with apparent HD who has <36 CAG repeats should be reported in the medical literature. Physicians should use particular caution in counseling individuals whose CAG repeat numbers fall in the intermediate range; we feel that there is more potential to over-estimate or over-emphasize the risk that such individuals will develop the disease or pass it on, than to under-estimate the problem. Referral to a skilled genetic counselor with detailed knowledge of HD genetics may be needed to help convey the current state of knowledge to the individual and their family.

CAG Repeat Number and Onset Age

There is a clear relationship between the CAG repeat number and the age at which HD symptoms begin, with the CAG repeat number explaining about 60-70% of the variation in onset age. Larger CAG repeat numbers are associated with younger disease onset ages. This relationship is not sufficiently uniform, however, to enable the physician to predict, based on the CAG repeat number alone, at what age a particular person will develop HD. In addition, knowledge of the CAG repeat number does not help the individual or physician to know what HD-related symptoms the person is going to develop or how severe they will be.

Meiotic Instability

While the CAG repeat numbers in a person's HD genes remain the same throughout his or her lifespan (at least in most clinically accessible tissues), the numbers may be different in the person's eggs or sperm. This is due to "meiotic instability," which refers to the tendency for CAG repeat numbers in the abnormal range to change as they pass through meiosis in the sperm and egg. Whereas normal CAG repeat numbers tend not to change much during meiosis, abnormally high CAG repeat numbers in the huntingtin gene tend to increase, but can decrease, as they are passed to the next generation. Thus, a child who inherits an abnormal HD gene from an affected parent ends up having a CAG repeat number in the abnormal gene that is not the same as the parent's CAG repeat number. For example, a parent passing on an HD gene that has 17 CAG repeats will likely have a child with 17 CAG repeats, but a parent passing on a 45 CAG repeat-containing gene is likely to have a child whose HD gene has 44, 46, 47, or more CAG repeats. The tendency for increases in CAG repeat number during meiosis are both more likely and greater in size when the abnormal HD gene is passed on by a father than a mother. This concept underlies three observations that were not well understood prior to the discovery of the HD gene: 1) the high proportion (up to 90% in some studies) of children with Juvenile onset HD who have an affected father; 2) "anticipation" - the earlier onset of symptoms in subsequent generations, and 3) "new mutations" for HD arising from a parent, usually a father, whose HD gene has a high-normal CAG repeat number.

Absent Family History of HD

About 5% of people who develop HD are unaware of any family history of the disease. This can sometimes be explained by early death of a gene-carrying parent, by adoption, or by mistaken paternity. However, others represent "new mutations," arising from the expansion of a parental CAG repeat number in the high-normal range (27-35 CAG repeats) during meiosis. Individuals with high normal CAG repeat sizes are not themselves at-risk for developing HD, but it is possible for those genes to manifest meiotic instability and lead to a child with a CAG repeat number in the abnormal range. We therefore refer to CAG repeat numbers from 27-35 as being in the "normal mutable range." Others use the less specific term, "intermediate range," as a synonym for "normal mutable range." The chance that someone with a CAG repeat number in the normal mutable range will have a child whose CAG repeat number is in the abnormal range cannot be predicted with accuracy; in research laboratories, an analysis of CAG repeat ranges in a sperm sample has been used to provide an empiric estimate of the risk in a specific individual, but it is not known whether the risk changes with advancing paternal age. Referral of these unusual cases to a genetic counselor who has experience in HD is recommended.

Genetic Testing

With the discovery of the HD gene in 1993, a simple and accurate genetic test became available. Genetic testing for HD is potentially useful in three clinical situations: diagnostic, or confirmatory testing; predictive, or presymptomatic testing; and prenatal testing.

The HD gene test usually requires a blood sample, but can be performed on other tissues, such as skin, amniocytes or chorionic villus cells, or autopsy material. The test requires special molecular diagnostic facilities, but at least two dozen university and commercial laboratories in North America perform gene tests for HD. A partial list of laboratories can be found at www.genetests.org, a nonprofit website that also contains useful information about many neurogenetic conditions. A list of genetic testing centers can also be found on the HDSA national web site, www.hdsa.org (click on "Living with HD" and then "genetic testing centers").

Diagnostic Testing

Diagnostic genetic testing refers to the use of a gene test in a person who has symptoms suggestive of HD, with or without a family history. If the clinical suspicion of HD is strong, this may be the only diagnostic test needed. It is important to remember that the presence of the huntingtin gene with an increased repeat number does not mean that a person's current symptoms are caused by HD, as the gene is present throughout life. Particularly in children, who cannot give informed consent, the gene test should be used only when the neurologic, cognitive or behavioral symptoms strongly suggest the onset and progression of HD.

Confirmatory testing should always be performed in a person who appears to have HD if no other affected family members have previously had a gene test, to be sure that the "family disease" is really HD and not some other condition. Diagnostic genetic testing should also be used routinely in an individual who appears to have HD but who has a negative or absent family history.

It is possible to make a clinical diagnosis of HD without a gene test. In fact, it is not the gene test, but the clinician, who determines that the symptoms of HD are present and how severe or disabling they are. This is a particularly important distinction when legal, financial, or other psychosocial decisions hinge on the presence of disabling symptoms caused by HD. A person's refusal to have a gene test should not prevent the physician from diagnosing HD, particularly if the person is from a known HD family.

Predictive Testing

Predictive testing refers to the use of an HD gene test in a person who has no symptoms but wants to know whether or not he carries the expanded gene. Predictive testing of healthy people requires a different clinical approach than the one to which neurologists are accustomed. There are no direct medical indications for, or benefits from, a predictive test. There are also potential psychosocial risks of predictive testing, including adverse effects on the individual's mood and self perception, on relationships with friends and family, and on insurability and employability. Predictive testing should be reserved for adults who have participated in a careful discussion with a genetic counselor about their genetic risks and the potential risks and benefits of the test itself.

Some people request predictive testing because they are concerned about symptoms that they, rightly or wrongly, have attributed to HD, but are afraid to ask about. Evaluation and treatment of symptoms should take precedence over predictive testing, to avoid the situation where the person's symptoms are incorrectly attributed to HD, and some other diagnosis is missed as a premature diagnosis of HD is made. A baseline neurologic exam and neuropsychological assessment prior to predictive testing can be helpful, but may lead to a clinical diagnosis of HD in a person who is not emotionally prepared to hear that he is currently symptomatic.

Physicians should seriously consider referring the interested at-risk individual to an HDSA genetic testing center or a genetic counselor for predictive testing, so that the person can receive pre-test counseling, accurate genetic information, and post-test support.

The Decision to Test and the Family

A special note should be made about the effects of a person's gene status on the entire family. The presence of an expanded HD gene in one individual has direct implications for that person's children, siblings, parents and collateral relatives. There may be family conflicts over the decision to test. Any physician who diagnoses HD, or who recommends a genetic test in one family member, must be prepared to face questions from and about these additional family members.

Results of predictive testing often weigh heavily on the caregiver or spouse. Therapy or counseling may be needed to help the caregiver cope with the test results.

The World Federation of Neurology, the International Huntington Association, and the Huntington's Disease Society of America have published guidelines regarding the genetic and psychological counseling and support that should surround predictive testing. In keeping with these guidelines, Huntington's Disease predictive testing centers have been established in various states. Referral of interested people to a predictive test center is highly recommended. A referral list of facilities offering predictive genetic testing for Huntington's Disease may be found on the HDSA national web site.

Care of the Person Who Has Had Predictive Testing

Although predictive genetic testing is often performed in conjunction with, or by, a genetics professional, it falls to the neurologist or primary care physician to follow the person who is known to be gene positive. This can be an awkward time for the physician, the person, and the family, who must find a middle ground between fatalism ("I already have HD and there's nothing to be done about it") and denial/ unawareness ("these symptoms aren't due to HD" or "I don't have any symptoms"). While most people cope well with the results of their gene test, there may be a need for ongoing counseling or support to help the individual adapt to his or her new status. If a baseline neurological examination was not performed as part of the predictive testing process, the gene-positive person should be encouraged to have a baseline exam, so that there are grounds for comparison later. Formal baseline neuropsychometric or neuropsychological assessment can also be very helpful.

Anyone touched by the outcome of genetic testing for HD may benefit from involvement with lay organization activities such as support groups, advocacy activities, and fundraising efforts, during this time of heightened awareness, anxiety and energy. Information on local support groups, HDSA Chapters and Affiliates can be found on the HDSA website, www.hdsa.org.

Research and Observational Trials

Participation in research is increasingly available to at-risk and gene-positive members of the HD community. Large observational studies such as PREDICT-HD, Registry, ENROLL-HD, and COHORT, are open to at-risk individuals, and are being performed at many sites in the U.S., Europe, and Latin America. Trials of potential therapeutic agents are also beginning at some sites. To find a list of current clinical and observational trials for HD in the U.S., go to www.hdsa.org, clinicaltrials.gov, or www.huntington-study-group.org.

Management of the At-risk Individual Who Has Not Had Predictive Testing

In the United States, the vast majority of at-risk individuals – 90% or more – do not undergo predictive testing. Some are concerned about the potential impact of genetic test results on insurability or employability (despite the recent passage of the Genetic Information Nondiscrimination Act, the intent of which is 1) to prevent health insurers from accessing genetic test information as part of their underwriting decision, and 2) to prevent employers from using genetic test results as part of employment decisions or processes). Some seem to have faith that researchers will find a treatment or cure for the disease in time for them; others may feel for one reason or another that they already "know" whether they are carriers or not, or that they could not emotionally handle the knowledge of their genetic fate. The majority of non-tested individuals, however, simply do not seem to seek this irreversible glimpse into the future.

Physicians must be able to provide predictive testing in a timely, private, and sensitive manner for those who desire it, while remaining respectful of the interests and concerns of those who do not. All at-risk individuals should be made aware that predictive testing is available, so that they can access it if they wish.

There is a potential for the at-risk individual to assign any and all symptoms to HD, and thereby miss out on appropriate evaluation of unrelated neurological or non-neurological health problems. Some at-risk individuals need emotional support as they deal with affected parents, anniversaries of difficult family events such as suicide, or as they make major life decisions about marriage, childbearing, or career choices. Genetic counseling about reproductive options should also be offered to at-risk individuals, whether or not they have previously undergone predictive testing.

At-risk individuals may also be ideal participants in HD community, advocacy, fundraising, and research efforts – often emerging as leaders of these efforts. Large-scale, world-wide observational studies such as COHORT, Registry, and ENROLL have expanded the opportunities for at-risk individuals to participate in research, including those who have not had a predictive gene test. Physicians can encourage people who are at-risk to become active members of the HD community. Local HDSA Chapters are a good resource for physician and at-risk individuals alike.

Reproductive Options and Prenatal Testing

Affected or at-risk individuals or couples should be informed of all of their reproductive options (shown in Table 1), with the understanding that different options are appropriate or desirable for different people. The discussion of reproductive options should be performed as part of overall genetic counseling and preferably before a pregnancy occurs.

For those who choose it, prenatal testing for HD can take several forms. One is pre-implantation genetic diagnostic testing (PGD), which is performed as part of an *in vitro* fertilization (IVF) procedure at specialized IVF centers. In this process, the woman uses fertility drugs so that she produces several oocytes at each cycle. The oocytes are fertilized with the partner's sperm, and the resulting embryos undergo genetic testing prior to implantation. Only an embryo with two normal HD genes is implanted, thus ensuring that the child will be free of the abnormal gene and will never develop HD or pass it on. IVF/PGD is performed at specialized centers, and is usually not covered by insurance.

Chorionic villus sampling is another form of prenatal testing, which may be performed very early, at 8-10 weeks after conception. Amniocentesis may also be used to obtain a sample for genetic testing at 14-16 weeks after conception. Tissue obtained through either procedure can be tested for the HD gene, with the option of termination of the pregnancy if the HD mutation is identified.

A non-disclosing prenatal genetic test can be performed, which determines only whether the fetus received a chromosome from the affected grandparent or the unaffected grandparent, without determining whether the fetus or at-risk parent actually carries the HD gene. This test requires samples from several people in the family and must be organized prior to the pregnancy.

Prenatal testing for HD is rarely requested in the United States, possibly because it includes consideration of a therapeutic abortion, which for many is not an option for religious, ethical, or psychological reasons, and possibly also because of the adult onset of symptoms.

A number of other reproductive options are available to couples in an HD family, including artificial insemination, adoption, surrogate mothers, or the decision to not reproduce. The genetic counselor can discuss each of the options shown in Table 1 without bias, so that the individual or couple can make the reproductive decision that is right for them.

TABLE 1: REPRODUCTIVE OPTIONS

- Natural reproduction without genetic testing
- Pre-implantation genetic diagnostic testing (PGD)
- Non-disclosing prenatal test
- Prenatal testing by amniocentesis or chorionic villus sampling
- Decision not to reproduce (may include sterilization)
- Artificial insemination
- Adoption
- Surrogate mother

Genetic Testing and the Prodrome of HD

The identification of the HD gene was a breakthrough in our understanding of how the disease is inherited and has made it possible for individuals to know if they carry the genetic mutation that causes HD. Given that currently there is no treatment which can slow, halt or reverse the disease, physicians should exercise caution in actively promoting predictive genetic testing. Furthermore, the presence or number of CAG repeats in the mutated HD gene does not indicate the age of onset. It is recommended that the physician refer at-risk individuals interested in predictive testing to a genetic counselor familiar with HD, as pre-test and post-test counseling can help the tested individual prepare for and manage their reaction to the results of the test.

The physician must also consider that the genetic test for HD can only confirm the presence of the gene and is not a means for clinical diagnosis of the onset of symptoms.

Observational studies underway are discovering tools for diagnosing the earliest changes caused by HD – changes which may occur 8-15 years before the onset of motor symptoms. MR imaging, neuropsychological tasks, and even neurological motor examination tasks, when performed under research protocols, can identify changes in gene-positive individuals long before the neurologist is able to diagnose the disease in the clinic. Researchers are beginning to use the terms "prodromal HD" or "pre-HD" to refer to the time when changes might be detectable with biochemical, imaging, or neuropsychological tests, but overt, clinically diagnosable HD has not yet developed.

It is not yet clear, though, how to apply these research findings to individuals in a clinical setting. Clinicians must, on the one hand, be available to treat symptoms as they occur in an at-risk person, and honest as to when they believe the disease is manifest and diagnosable, without leaping to a diagnosis of HD the first time a person experiences depression, or diagnosing manifest disease in an asymptomatic person based solely on an MRI scan.

During this era, where our ability to diagnose the disease is not yet matched by effective treatments, it will be the physician's challenge to provide honest information in a timely, yet sensitive manner and then work creatively with the individual to manage symptoms and maintain quality of life.

Case Study: #1

Genetic Counseling and Genetic Testing: Predictive Testing for Reproductive Reasons

A 25 year old woman comes to her father's appointment. She asks the doctor how she can get a gene test. She is married and has a number of career and family decisions coming up for which she thinks knowledge of her gene status would be important. She is referred to an HD genetic testing center.

She speaks to the genetic counselor, who recommends that she establish whatever health, life, disability, and long-term care insurance she wants, prior to setting her first in-person appointment. The counselor also recommends that she bring her husband with her to her pre-test appointments, which is a problem, as she has not informed her husband that she is at-risk for HD.

The woman comes alone to her first appointment, where the genetics of HD are discussed, as well as the potential impact of the results on her and her family. Misunderstandings about the genetics of HD are corrected. The woman is next scheduled to see the psychologist. She admits that she had always thought that she would probably not get HD because all the affected people in her family are male. It was because of this belief that she had not spoken to her husband about her at-risk status. The psychologist recommends that they bring her husband into the discussion before proceeding with the testing process.

One year later, the woman returns to have a predictive test. She has spoken to her husband and he is willing to provide support during the testing process. She wishes to participate in an HD research study if she tests positive, and whatever the test result, is hoping to start a family soon. After speaking with the genetic counselor and the neurologist, she has blood drawn, and a results visit is scheduled three weeks later.

Together, the neurologist and genetic counselor present the results, which unfortunately confirm that the woman has the mutation responsible for HD. The woman accept the results, remains interested in participating in research and is considering IVF with preimplantation genetic diagnosis.

Genetic Counseling and Genetic Testing: Predictive Testing and the Family

A 30 year old woman called the clinic to request predictive testing for HD. Her 40 year old sister had recently been diagnosed with HD, and their brother had undergone predictive testing elsewhere. When told that the predictive testing center listed on the HDSA website provided predictive testing in a context of genetic counseling, a psychological assessment and a neurologic examination, the woman became very angry, indicating that her brother's doctor had just sent a blood sample to the laboratory and called him with the results, and that she already knew everything that a genetic counselor could tell her.

The clinic's genetic counselor spoke to her on the phone, and encouraged her to establish health, life, disability and long-term care insurance (if desired) prior to completing her predictive test, and to consider whether she wanted to self-pay for testing-related services or submit them to her insurance company. During later in-person visits, the genetic aspects of HD were reviewed, and several misconceptions clarified. Her neurologic examination was normal, which surprised her, as she was concerned about headaches and insomnia, and mistakenly thought they were caused by HD.

After she learned more about the genetic aspects of the disease, she realized that her brother's result was in the "indeterminate range," and she brought him to the clinic so that they could review the clinical relevance of his result with her neurologist.

The results of her gene test showed two normal genes. The woman was very pleased with the results, and in retrospect, glad that she had undergone a neurologic examination and now understood more about the genetic aspects of HD. She indicated her intent to help her brother through his disease course, now that she knew that she would be unaffected. She was invited to participate, along with her family, in the COHORT (observational) study. A few months later, she called the genetic counselor; she was in a serious relationship, and wanted to be reassured that her biological children would not be at-risk for HD. The genetic counselor reassured her that, as a carrier of two normal genes, she could only pass normal genes onto her children.

Chapter 3

Team Care for
Huntington's Disease

Martha Nance, M.D.

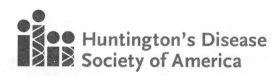
Huntington's Disease
Society of America

Team Care for Huntington's Disease

Huntington's Disease (HD) is a neurological, psychiatric, and genetic disease that progresses slowly over years, even decades. Optimal care for this complex disease requires a team of health professionals, as well as a network of supportive daily caregivers, including family, friends or professional aides. No one doctor or one caregiver should attempt to manage all aspects of an HD case without assistance.

HDSA has established 21 HDSA Centers of Excellence around the country, where multidisciplinary teams of specialists partner with families to manage symptoms, reduce complications, identify resources for support, prepare for the future, and receive genetic and psychological counseling. Not everyone lives near a HDSA Center of Excellence, however, and there are families who prefer to have their loved one's care overseen by a trusted family doctor.

The purpose of this chapter is to help the interested physician to understand how allied health professionals can complement his expertise, so that the person with HD can receive excellent care within or outside of the designated HDSA Centers of Excellence. A listing of the Centers and contact information for the sites is provided on the HDSA website at www.hdsa.org and in Appendix III of this handbook, the Resource Directory.

The Concept of Team-Based Care

The care-defining characteristics of HD are shown in Table 1.

Table 1. Care-defining characteristics of HD
Adult-onset (usually)
Genetic disorder
Movement disorder
Psychiatric/behavioral disorder
Changing mental function
Degenerative (progressive) over years
Purely neurologic disorder (spares other organs)
Fatal

HD primarily affects the brain, and is therefore often managed by a neurologist, particularly one who specializes in movement disorders (in the discussion below, we will define the neurologist as the primary managing physician, which is the case at most HDSA Centers of Excellence). However, it is certainly possible for a thoughtful primary care practitioner to fill this role.

Because many people with HD exhibit moderate to severe neurobehavioral symptoms, the neurologist may work in coordination with a psychiatrist or psychologist. Caregivers and other family members may also benefit from family counseling or grief counseling by a psychologist. A neuropsychologist can provide periodic assessments of changing mental function, help the affected individual to make the most of their current abilities and help families to adapt to the increasing deficiencies.

HD progresses over many years and primary care will be needed throughout the course of the disease to address the general health concerns of the individual. For example, dental care, including annual dental checkups, will help to maintain good speech and swallowing function for as long as possible.

Genetic counseling and testing is another aspect of HD that may be unfamiliar to the managing physician or neurologist. Decisions surrounding genetic testing in an HD family may be extremely complex and emotional (see Chapter 2, Genetic Testing) and it is recommended that an interested HD person or family member be referred to a geneticist or genetic counselor for these aspects of individual and family management.

The physician, as team leader, will develop a long-term relationship with people with HD in his care and their families, which can extend over generations. This relationship can be interesting and rewarding. We believe that, given the absence of a cure for this difficult disease, helping people to live their lives to the fullest and to die comfortably when the time comes, is a demonstration of medicine at its best.

The HD Care Team

The goals of treatment for HD are to reduce the burden of symptoms, maximize function and optimize quality of life. Various health professionals may be needed to achieve these goals and the care team will fluctuate in number and area of expertise over time, as the individual's symptoms progress and change through the course of the disease.

Health Professional	Role in HD Care
Neurologist	Overall care coordination ("team leader"); neurological management
Psychiatrist	Overall care coordination ("team leader"): psychiatric management
Psychologist	Counseling about relationships, grief, chronic disease, symptom management, etc.; family support
Neuropsychologist	Neuropsychological assessment and counseling about cognitive changes
Geneticist or Genetic counselor	Genetic counseling, predictive testing, prenatal or preimplantation genetic testing
Social worker	Disability, financial planning, management of social crises, accessing community services, placement outside the home; Advance Directives; counseling (if licensed)
Physical therapy	Gait assessment and assistive devices; exercise program
Occupational therapy	Assessment of driving, home safety, and activities of daily living; equipment for seating, feeding, hygiene, etc.
Speech therapy	Speech assessment, alternative communication devices; dysphagia assessment and counseling
Dietician	Nutritional assessment and counseling
Nursing	Case management, telephone counseling, support
Research team	Counseling about research opportunities; enrollment in research
Chaplain	Family support, spiritual advice
Lay organization volunteer	Liaison with HD support groups, advocacy, other organization activities
Primary care physician	Primary care, preventive health, management of medical complications in late stages
Dentist	Aggressive, proactive dental care
Hospice care team	Comfort- and dignity-directed care in terminal stages

The table on page 29 shows the variety of health professionals who may have a role to play in the care of the person with HD. Managing physicians may have to seek local specialists in these areas who are willing to take on the challenges that HD presents.

Typical Healthcare Team at an HDSA Center of Excellence

Primary
- Neurologist
- Psychiatrist/psychologist
- Neuropsychiatrist/neuropsychologist
- Genetic counselor
- Social worker
- Clinic coordinator
- Nursing

Ancillary
- Physical therapist
- Occupational therapist
- Speech-language pathologist
- Dietician

Other
- Research coordinator
- Chaplain

Principles of HD Management

Treating HD can be frustrating for the physician, the caregiver and the person with HD as there are few pharmacologic therapies of proven benefit. However, there is always something the physician can do to reduce the burden of symptoms. For example, the physician can ensure that a speech-language pathologist has evaluated swallowing and made appropriate recommendations to reduce the risk of choking, ascertain if the person with HD has completed an Advance Directives form, or, during the terminal stage of the disease, ensure that any pain is well managed and that all appropriate hospice services are being utilized.

Rather than feeling handicapped by a lack of proven pharmacotherapies, creative physicians and allied health professionals can use common sense and experience to develop care strategies to ease symptoms and help family members use their own creativity to optimize function and quality of life. Personnel at HDSA Centers of Excellence around the country are uniformly willing to assist physicians and other allied health professionals to address the many challenges that HD presents.

Team Care as HD Progresses

People with HD and their families can face the challenges of the disease more effectively if they know ahead of time what is coming. This does not mean focusing on the terminal aspects of the disease. HD develops over many years, and affected individuals may live in late stage HD for up to a decade. The physician, as leader of the care team, must keep the focus on maintaining the person's quality of life throughout the course of the disease.

The chart on page 31 illustrates how the varied health professionals can contribute to improving the life of the person with HD.

Typical Contributions of Care Team Members during the Different Stages of HD

Health professional	Stage 1-2 (Early)	Stage 3 (Middle)	Stage 4-5 (Late)
Neurologist	Diagnosis, overall care coordination, neurological management, referrals to other team members		
Psychiatrist	Overall care coordination; psychiatric management: medications, navigating mental health care system		
Psychologist	Relationship counseling; grief in chronic disease; child/adolescent counseling; non-pharmacologic approaches to anxiety, depression, stress, etc.	Caregiver support; behavioral management	Family support related to grief and dying
Neuropsychologist	Neuropsychological assessment; counseling person about compensatory strategies; assessment of disability, driving capacity	Neuropsychological assessment as needed; assessment of competence; counseling family about cognitive changes	
Geneticist or Genetic counselor	Genetic counseling, predictive testing, prenatal or preimplantation genetic testing	Counseling of family members, such as children	
Social worker	Disability; financial, insurance planning; management of social crises; information about support groups, HD programs; psychosocial counseling (if licensed)	Advance Directives; accessing community services (e.g. Meals on Wheels, day programs, transportation services)	Advance Directives, if not already in place; respite care, community services, placement outside the home; managing family conflicts
Physical therapy	Exercise program, home preparedness and safety	Gait assessment, assistive devices; home safety	Non-pharmacologic management of dystonia
Occupational therapy	Workplace assessment if appropriate; assessment of driving skills	Home safety, equipment, and services; assessment of ADLs	Equipment for seating, sleeping, feeding, hygiene, etc.
Speech therapy	Pre-emptive evaluation of swallow function, counseling about safe swallowing	Re-evaluate dysphagia; individual and family counseling as needed; reassessment of speech and communication	Re-evaluate dysphagia; diet texture modification; simple communication devices or systems
Dietician	Nutritional assessment; general "healthy eating in HD" recommendations	Assist speech therapy in food texture recommendations; supplements if weight loss is present	Calorie counts, food recommendations; altered food and liquid textures; assist with proper feeding tube supplements if appropriate
Nursing	Case management, telephone counseling, support for individual and family		
Research team	Counseling about research opportunities; enrollment in research studies	Enrollment in research studies	
Chaplain	Individual and family spiritual support; assist with decisions about Advance Directives, Hospice		
Lay organization volunteer	Liaison with HD support groups, advocacy, other organization activities; coordinate with health professionals to identify support group facilitators (e.g. social worker or genetic counselor)		
Primary care physician	Primary care, ordinary preventive health measures (mammography, colonoscopy, vaccinations, management of other chronic diseases, etc.)	Ordinary primary care	Management of typical medical complications: vitamin deficiencies, skin breakdown, bursitis, fractures, urinary and pulmonary infections; liaise with Hospice team
Dentist	Aggressive, proactive dental care		
Hospice care team			Comfort- and dignity-focused care in terminal stages

Summary

HD is a disease well-suited to team-based care, many components of which should be available in any medical community. HDSA Centers of Excellence can provide information, referrals and backup to the physician. The goal of team care, which is clearly achievable, is to relieve symptoms, maximize function and optimize the quality of life throughout the person's course with HD.

Case Study: #1

Team Care for HD: Improving Care and Quality of Life

A 36 year old man and his wife come to the neurologist to establish care for his Huntington's Disease. His diagnosis was made three years earlier. He had recently been fired from his factory assembly job because of suspicion of drunkenness. Although he denied any significant symptoms, his wife noted that he was irritable, slept poorly, and was obsessive about his bowel movements, spending hours in the bathroom every day. He had moderate chorea, moderate dysarthria, motor impersistence, and gait instability. He had lost 15 pounds over the previous six months.

The man was started on an SSRI for his obsessive/perseverative behaviors, and a low dose of neuroleptic drug at bedtime to reduce irritability and obsessiveness, and to stabilize sleep (neither have FDA approval for use in HD). He was referred for formal neuropsychological assessment, and met with the social worker to assist with the completion of disability forms. A speech-language pathologist evaluated his swallow function, which was minimally impaired, and the dietician discussed his caloric needs and made recommendations about high calorie foods and nutritional supplements. The man and his wife had not previously met with a genetic counselor, so a genetics consultation was arranged. The physical therapist recommended a daily exercise program to help the man maintain his mobility and balance.

The man's wife was struggling with the situation, as she was also working part-time and caring for the couple's two children. The social worker recommended local support groups, reputable websites, and also recommended a psychologist familiar with family issues in HD. They were encouraged to apply for benefits from Social Security Disability Insurance (SSDI), as it appeared that it was the neurologic disease that was interfering with the husband's ability to work at a competitive job.

A follow-up appointment with the doctor was scheduled for one month later, to evaluate the effects of medication changes and ensure that the recommendations of the health team had been well-received. At that time, the man's wife reported that his irritability was improved, and that he was sleeping better, although he was still somewhat perseverative. They were interested in enrolling in an HD research study, and were planning to go to a support group meeting the following month.

Case Study: #2

Team Care in HD: Diagnosis

A 35 year old woman comes to the clinic with her parents. She was adopted and nothing was known of her birth parents. At age 32, she had developed anxiety and depression. After a variety of relationship, financial, and legal problems, she visited a psychiatrist, who referred her to a neurologist because of some involuntary movements. This neurologist attributed the movements to the use of risperidone as a mood stabilizer, ordered an MRI scan that was interpreted as "normal," and prescribed benztropine for her tremors. The family physician found no evidence of medical disease, despite the woman's rapid 15 pound weight loss.

Suspecting Huntington's Disease, her family made an appointment at the nearest HDSA Center of Excellence. The neurologist there found abnormal involuntary movements, abnormal saccadic eye movements, impersistence of tongue protrusion, inability to perform a three-step motor command, diffusely brisk reflexes, and an erratic lurching gait. Because the history and examination were consistent with a diagnosis of HD, formal neuropsychometric testing and a diagnostic HD gene test were ordered. A review of the previous MRI showed subtle caudate atrophy and mild brain atrophy, abnormal for the woman's age. No new medications were needed, as the depression and anxiety were, by then, adequately controlled, but benztropine was deemed to be unnecessary and was discontinued.

When the gene test results confirmed the diagnosis of HD, the clinical features, genetic aspects, and typical course of HD were reviewed with the woman and her family. A swallow evaluation with the speech-language pathologist was ordered. The social worker spoke with the family about applying for Social Security Disability Insurance benefits, as the psychometric testing showed moderate subcortical dementia. The dietician talked with the woman and her family about healthy eating and strategies to increase caloric intake. The woman was invited to participate in a clinical research trial of a novel HD treatment, and invited to the next meeting of an HD support group.

Six months later, she had successfully qualified for Social Security Disability Insurance benefits, and had moved into an assisted living facility near her parents. She had completed her Advance Care Directives, and was an active participant in a clinical research study. She had also become involved in volunteer HDSA Chapter advocacy efforts. Her mood had brightened substantially as she now understood the cause of her disabilities.

Special Topic

Driving Cessation in HD

Adam Rosenblatt, M.D.

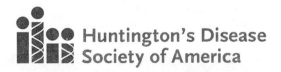

Driving Cessation in HD

The assessment of safety to drive is a crucial duty of the clinician who works with people with Huntington's Disease (HD). It is complicated by four factors: difficulties in predicting driving abilities in an office setting, the importance of driving for maintaining independence and self-esteem, the lack of insight about their driving impairment found in many persons with HD, and the reluctance of family members to enforce a restriction which they know will be a severe blow to their loved one. Nevertheless, we know of several traffic fatalities affecting both people with HD and bystanders, caused by drivers with HD, some of whom had already been warned.

The issue of driving safety should be discussed periodically with any person with manifest HD and their family. Sometimes the person with HD has already begun to limit driving, such as by not driving at night, or in bad weather, in unfamiliar areas, or on crowded high speed roads. In fact, in the majority of cases in our experience, people with HD stop driving at the appropriate time without any significant arguments or need for coercion. Those who have not stopped driving fit into one of three categories: Those with no discernable problems, those who represent an obvious menace, usually because of a record of prior incidents or grossly impaired judgment, and those about whom the clinician is initially unsure. Unfortunately this last group is the largest in any typical practice.

Clinicians facing this issue may be guided by the answers to some broad questions: Has the person with HD already been in some recent accidents or received traffic citations? Uninsightful or desperate individuals may not always be upfront about these issues, and the family can be encouraged to examine the car for dents and scratches and to make sure the insurer has not cancelled the person's policy. Have friends or family members observed the person's driving or ridden in the car while the person with HD was driving? Have they noticed any irregularities such as swerving, errors of judgment, difficulty braking, or uneven pressure on the accelerator? Do they consider the person to be a safe driver? A good rule of thumb is that if a person's family would not allow him to pick up children from school then he does not belong on the road. Family members may fear the person's reaction to their opinions and should be given a chance to speak to the physician alone. They may need advice and support to help them feel strong enough to take the necessary steps.

In less obvious cases, it can be difficult to assess driving safety in a clinic or office setting, and physicians may wish to refer some people with HD for formal assessments, usually administered by occupational therapists, and available at some hospitals and rehabilitation facilities. Nevertheless, even these programs may not get at the issue of judgment or performance under stress, that is, a person with HD may "pass" an evaluation under tightly controlled conditions, but still be unsafe on the road.

The person with HD and their family must also be reminded that HD is a progressive disease and that driving will need to be re-evaluated frequently even if it does not present an immediate problem. Individuals and families should be encouraged to think ahead and develop a plan for driving cessation that addresses questions such as "Is the person living in an accessible area? Where does the person have to go on a regular basis? Can other neighbors, friends, and family provide rides? Is there public transportation or van service available? Are their community programs available for the disabled?"

When a physician advises a person with HD to stop driving, the instruction should be presented in a caring and supportive way, emphasizing the doctor's and family's concern for the person's safety and their certainty that the person would not want to hurt anyone else because of impaired driving. The doctor should remind the person with HD that she may not always be able to see the manifestations of the disease in herself, but that the recommendation is being made on the basis of the person's history up to this point, observations in the clinic, and information from outside sources. It may be helpful to explain that the doctor worries that the person with HD may not commit a driving error herself, but might not be able to avoid an accident due to slowed reaction time in a situation such as another driver running a stop sign, or a child chasing a ball into the street. Once a person with HD makes the difficult decision to stop driving, the clinic, family, friends and neighbors should acknowledge the person's honorable behavior and marshal their forces in support, by providing rides, company, financial help, and assistance with errands, and by looking into community programs which may offer extra support to those who can no longer drive.

Sometimes the physician may wish to minimize family discord by "playing the heavy" and instructing the person with HD to stop driving, emphasizing his or her own observations and the overall severity of HD symptoms without making the family's report the focus of the conversation, but this needs to be discussed explicitly with the family so that they will support the decision. In life and death matters such as this, the instruction to stop driving is not a recommendation. It is a doctor's order. The physician must be willing to expend considerable emotional goodwill on this issue or even to lose the person from her practice entirely. A recalcitrant individual should be told that the assessment of him as an unsafe driver and the explicit instruction to stop will be entered into his permanent medical record, and that the doctor will not support him if an accident occurs. In especially problematic cases it may be necessary to have the person's license suspended over his objections, or even to have the car impounded.

The doctor's responsibility regarding unsafe drivers will vary by state, province or country. In some municipalities, physicians are obligated to report individuals who are unsafe to drive because of certain medical conditions or unsafe drivers in general. In other areas, to do so would constitute a breach of doctor/patient confidentiality. Family members do not owe the person with HD confidentiality and may be encouraged in such cases to make the report themselves, or with very impaired individuals, to remove or disable the car. Confidentiality is not an absolute right, and it is sometimes trumped by a physician's duty to the life and safety of the individual and the safety of the public. When there is no other alternative, it may be necessary for a physician to deliberately breach confidentiality to report a person's behavior to the authorities. In such a case the doctor should seek legal consultation, document the case carefully, and inform the family and person with HD that he is doing so.

Chapter 4

The Motor Disorder

Vicki Wheelock, M.D.

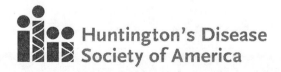
Huntington's Disease
Society of America

The Motor Disorder

Movement-associated symptoms are a core feature of Huntington's Disease (HD). The most recognized motor symptom is chorea, but a number of additional movement disorders occur, including dystonia, bradykinesia, rigidity, myoclonus, tics, and tremor. Moreover, people with HD experience a progressive loss of control of voluntary movement, resulting in functional decline and increasing dependence. Early motor symptoms may be quite subtle and mild, but as HD progresses virtually all movement-associated functions are affected, including finger dexterity and hand coordination, gait, and speech and swallowing function. Additional late stage challenges include bowel and bladder incontinence, moderate to severe weight loss, and pain. While disease modifying therapies are not yet available, a number of effective treatments exist for symptomatic management. These treatments improve quality of life and can reduce caregiver burden.

Presenting Symptoms by Age of Onset

Age at onset commonly determines the initial cluster of motor symptoms experienced by the individual with HD. Juvenile onset HD is characterized by rigidity, bradykinesia, dystonia, and sometimes tremor and myoclonus tremors. Chorea is typically absent (see Chapter 7, Juvenile onset HD).

Adult-onset HD may be initially characterized by chorea, progressing later to dystonia and rigidity. About 10% of adults with HD present with an akinetic-rigid form of HD, with predominant dystonia and a paucity of chorea.

Chorea

More than 90% of people affected by HD have chorea. Chorea is characterized by involuntary movements which are often sudden, irregular and purposeless or semi-purposeful. The movements are often more prominent in the extremities early in the disease, but may eventually include facial grimacing, eyelid elevation, neck, shoulder, trunk, and leg movements as the disease progresses. Mild chorea can be voluntarily suppressed, but re-emerges when the person with HD is distracted. Chorea typically increases in frequency and amplitude over time, and may peak about 10 years after disease onset. In some people, chorea then plateaus and lessens, while others have inexorable worsening as they enter late stage HD.

In early HD, chorea may be difficult for the clinician to detect during the office visit. Because involuntary movements may cease at the start of the physical examination, the physician should take note of their presence while obtaining the history. When a history of involuntary movements is not confirmed during the examination, it may be helpful to observe the person with HD during mental distraction tasks such as counting backward.

Rating Chorea

Assessing chorea, before and after treatment with a medication, is often done using the Unified Huntington's Disease Rating Scale (UHDRS), a research tool which has been developed by the Huntington Study Group (HSG) to provide a uniform assessment of the clinical features and course of HD. The UHDRS has undergone extensive reliability and validity testing and has been used as a major outcome measure by the HSG in controlled clinical trials. Information on obtaining the entire

UHDRS may be found on the HSG website, www.huntington-study-group.org, by clicking on the Resources tab.

The UHDRS includes a subscale for assessing motor disorders. Chorea is rated in one of seven body regions. The total chorea score is the sum of the scores for each body region, and can range from 0 – 28.

Unified Huntington's Disease Rating Scale Motor Assessment Chorea Scale		
Body Region	Severity	
Face	0	Absent
Bucco-oral-lingual	1	Slight/intermittent
Trunk	2	Mild/common or moderate/intermittent
Right upper extremity	3	Moderate/common
Left upper extremity	4	Marked/prolonged
Right lower extremity	Total score: Sum of scores for each body region Range = 0 - 28	
Left lower extremity		

Symptoms of chorea can range from absent to severe. Chorea in the legs may result in a lurching gait, sometimes with brief flexion of the knees. People with HD are commonly unaware of mild chorea and may not require pharmacological treatment for the condition.

Social embarrassment or sleep interruption may occur as chorea increases. Individuals who have mild chorea that primarily limits sleep may benefit from low-dose long-acting benzodiazepines such as diazepam or clonazepam at bedtime.

Moderate to severe chorea can cause pain, repeated injury, falls, and poor sleep. Facial and bucco-oro-lingual chorea can lead to repeated tongue and lip injuries, impairing nutritional status and hydration. Individuals with severe chorea develop a downward spiral with pain, tissue injury, weight loss, difficulty concentrating and communicating, and growing dependence on caregivers. They may require helmets and protective padding to prevent injury. Adaptive chairs, toilet seats, low beds, and padding of the environment can be helpful in the home or in the long-term care facility. An occupational therapist can help the family identify suppliers of equipment, and to consider other safety issues within and outside the home.

Chorea increases with stress and anxiety. Strategies to reduce chorea include stress reduction and management of mood disorders. Having the caregiver set up routines and schedules that allow extra time for dressing, hygiene, meals and daily activities can be helpful.

Symptoms that indicate the need for possible pharmacologic management of chorea include muscle pain, frequent dropping of items, repetitive injuries, falls associated with chorea of the trunk and limbs, poor sleep, and weight loss. Individuals with a total chorea score of 10 or greater may be candidates for pharmacologic treatment. Some people with HD, with milder chorea, who are nonetheless very symptomatic may also benefit from treatment.

Treatment of Chorea

In 2008 the Food and Drug Administration approved tetrabenazine (Xenazine®) for the relief of chorea in Huntington's Disease. Tetrabenazine is a highly effective treatment, reducing the total chorea score by 5 points in a double-blind, placebo controlled trial. The mechanism of action is depletion of dopamine release by presynaptic striatal neurons. Side effects include sedation, depression, akathisia, and worsening of voluntary motor control. About 20% of individuals in the placebo-controlled trial experienced new onset or worsening of depression, and there was one completed suicide. Physicians must discuss this risk with individuals and their caregivers, and clinical monitoring must be provided. In addition, the FDA requires that tetrabenazine be released through a centralized mail-order pharmacy system.

Tetrabenazine may prolong the corrected QT interval (QTc), and caution is advised when used in combination with other drugs or medical conditions that potentially prolong the QTc. Physicians are also cautioned about the potential risk of tardive dyskinesia or neuroleptic malignant syndrome, although neither occurred in the 12-week randomized trial.

The initial dose of tetrabenazine is 12.5 mg daily, increasing weekly by 12.5 mg in 2-3 divided doses per day up to 50 mg/day. The principle of "starting low and going slow" with dose titration helps determine the lowest effective dose and reduces unwanted side effects. For milder chorea, a dose of 12.5 mg twice daily may be effective, with higher doses reserved for more difficult chorea. In the double-blind study, doses of 50 mg/day were as effective as higher doses, but in people with severe chorea, higher doses may be necessary. The dose of tetrabenazine should be halved for people with HD who are also taking strong CYP2D6 inhibitors such as fluoxetine, paroxetine and quinidine. The FDA recommends CYP2D6 genotyping for individuals who require a dose of > 50 mg/day in order to identify fast- and slow-metabolizers. More details on testing can be provided by calling 1-888-882-6013.

Individuals who do not tolerate tetrabenazine, or have other contraindications to its use, may benefit from off-label use of neuroleptics for reduction in chorea. Neuroleptics block dopamine at the striatal post-synaptic receptor. Typical neuroleptics such as haloperidol or fluphenazine are quite effective. Some atypical neuroleptics such as olanzapine and risperidone may also be effective. The atypical neuroleptics, quetiapine and clozapine, do not block dopamine D2 receptors and are generally ineffective for chorea. Side effects of neuroleptics include apathy, sedation, akathisia, worsening of voluntary motor control, tardive dyskinesia and neuroleptic malignant syndrome. Additional side effects of atypical neuroleptics include weight gain and metabolic syndrome. However, this tendency to weight gain can be beneficial in an individual with HD who has severe chorea accompanied by severe weight loss.

Medication	Initial dose	Maximal dose	Side effects
Tetrabenazine	12.5 mg	50 mg/day	Depression, Akathisia, Worsening of voluntary motor control, Sedation
Haloperidol	0.5 – 1 mg	10 – 15 mg/day	Extrapyramidal syndrome (abnormal involuntary movements): Akathisia, dystonia, bradykinesia Sedation
Fluphenazine	1 – 2 mg	10 mg/day	Extrapyramidal syndrome Sedation
Risperidone	0.5 – 1 mg	5 – 10 mg/day	Extrapyramidal syndrome at higher doses Sedation
Olanzapine	1.25 – 2.5 mg	10 – 15 mg/day	Extrapyramidal syndrome Sedation Weight gain and metabolic syndrome

Individuals who require anti-chorea therapy and have co-morbid behavioral/psychiatric disorders (psychosis, episodic aggression and agitation not managed by behavioral interventions, or bipolar disorder) may also be better managed by neuroleptic medications rather than tetrabenazine.

Anti-chorea therapy should be re-evaluated at least annually. Some individuals will require increasing doses of anti-chorea medications over time. Many will eventually develop increasing dystonia and rigidity with HD progression, necessitating reduction or cessation of anti-chorea medications.

Dystonia

Dystonia is characterized by a repetitive, abnormal pattern of muscle contraction frequently associated with a twisting quality. Examples of dystonia in HD include dystonic arm elevation while walking, tilting of the trunk, bruxism, or elevation and adduction of the foot while walking. These postures and movements may be quite asymmetric. Dystonia often emerges in mid to late stage HD, but it is quite common in juvenile and the adult-onset rigid-dystonic variant of HD. Trunk dystonia may, at times, be an early symptom and can cause significant back pain.

Pharmacologic treatment of dystonia in HD may include benzodiazepines, baclofen, and sometimes dopaminergic agents developed for Parkinson's disease. Botulinum toxin injections can be quite effective for focal dystonias. Careful monitoring for hallucinations and psychosis is necessary when using dopaminergic agents. Some people with HD, with severe dystonia, benefit from braces, pads, or splints for affected joints; a physical or occupational therapist can assist in the evaluation and dispensing of appropriate equipment.

Bradykinesia

Bradykinesia implies slowing of automatic or voluntary movements. Loss of facial expressivity, absence of arm swing, difficulty with finger tapping and rapid alternating movements and gait slowness are quite common, and worsen with disease progression. Bradykinesia may coexist with, but be difficult to recognize in the presence of additional hyperkinetic findings of chorea and dystonia. Anti-chorea therapy may unmask or worsen bradykinesia. Bradykinesia in people with Juvenile onset HD, and adults with the rigid/dystonic form of HD, may improve with treatment with amantadine or carbidopa/levodopa. As noted above, careful monitoring for hallucinations and psychosis is recommended when these agents are used.

Other Movement Disorders in HD

Tics are sudden, brief, intermittent movements, gestures or vocalizations that mimic fragments of normal behavior. Respiratory and vocal tics can produce sniffs, grunts, moans or coughs. If severe, they can be reduced by benzodiazepines, SSRIs, neuroleptics and possibly by off-label use of tetrabenazine.

Myoclonus is characterized by sudden, brief, shock-like involuntary movements. Tremor is a rhythmic oscillating movement present at rest, with posture, or with voluntary movements. Myoclonus and tremor are much more commonly seen in Juvenile onset HD or in young adults. Clonazepam is quite effective. A resting parkinsonian tremor may appear as a side effect of neuroleptic therapy for psychosis or chorea in persons with HD. Neuroleptic drug dose reduction or change to an atypical agent should be considered.

Rigidity, which is characterized by an increase in muscle tone and a reduction of passive range of motion, may occur early in juvenile or adult akinetic/rigid HD, but is also common in advanced HD. Rigidity may be improved by reduction or cessation of tetrabenazine or neuroleptic drugs, or by benzodiazepines, baclofen and possibly by dopaminergic drugs.

Impaired Voluntary Motor Control

Progressive loss of voluntary motor control is a core feature of HD. This symptom starts early in the disease, progresses inexorably, and correlates with disability. Slow initiation and velocity of saccadic eye movements are early signs of voluntary movement impairment. Difficulty with finger and manual dexterity are also encountered as early signs. People with HD experience clumsiness and awkwardness in carrying out manual tasks. Initial exam findings may include slowness in finger tapping and rapid alternating movements of the hands. As the disease progresses, finger tapping becomes more irregular and arrests in movement appear. In late stage, people with HD lose the ability to perform most voluntary movements. They are often mute, akinetic, rigid, and dystonic, with hyper reflexia and extensor plantar reflexes.

Motor impersistence is the inability to maintain voluntary motor contraction. Symptoms may include the "milk-maid's grip" or uneven pressure on the gas pedal while driving. Motor impersistence steadily worsens as HD progresses. This difficulty may lead to dropping items, difficulty with writing and manual tasks, and may even prevent the effective use of a walker. Clinical testing for motor impersistence includes sustained maximum eyelid closure or tongue protrusion. Unfortunately, there are no medications that improve motor control in HD.

Gait Impairment and Falls

Gait impairment and falls typically occur in mid to late stage HD. The gait gradually becomes slower and more wide-based. Chorea and dystonia of the trunk and legs can contribute to gait disturbances and falls. Dramatic changes in posture occasionally occur, with trunk dystonia or chorea leading to significant postural perturbations. Postural reflexes become impaired, with falls occurring when the center of gravity is displaced. Early referral to a physical therapist for gait assessment, balance and postural exercises is strongly recommended.

As gait difficulties increase, the use of proper footwear and adaptive equipment should be encouraged. Deluxe 4-wheeled walkers with handbrakes are often quite effective in stabilizing gait, but cognitive difficulties or loss of manual dexterity may prevent effective use of walkers for some people with HD. When these measures fail, a transition to using a wheelchair for safety is indicated. Some individuals may be able to self-propel in a standard wheelchair using their arms and legs. Those with difficult chorea or trunk dystonia may benefit from a custom wheelchair with a reclining back, elevating leg rests, removable armrests and a pommel ("saddle") seat to prevent sliding out.

Speech Impairment

Dysarthria is another frequent symptom of motor dysfunction in HD. The rhythm and speed of speech changes with bursts of words alternating with pauses. Speech becomes slower, and with disease progression, the voice may become hypophonic or explosive. Articulation of speech becomes impaired when voluntary control of lips, tongue and mouth declines. The coordination of speaking and breathing declines, and the intelligibility of speech deteriorates. Delays in initiation of speech, paucity of speech, and finally mutism occur. Referral to a speech-language pathologist may be indicated when articulation or intelligibility is affected. Motor dyscontrol or cognitive dysfunction often prevents the person with HD from using keyboard- or computer-based augmentative communication devices successfully. However, simple "word boards" placed on the lap can help some people with HD to communicate simple ideas and questions. Caregivers should be educated about behavioral strategies to improve communication. Please refer to the discussion in Chapter 5, under *Language*.

Swallow Dysfunction and Choking

Dysphagia is a common symptom in HD. The automatic coordination of bringing food to the mouth, chewing, forming a bolus and swallowing, while simultaneously inhibiting breathing, breaks down. Food may spill from the mouth. People with HD may inadequately chew foods, and commonly add more mouthfuls of food before swallowing. Poor coordination may lead to frequent choking on liquids and on solid food. Aspiration of liquids or food may lead to pneumonia or even to death by choking.

A speech-language pathologist should assess the individual with dysphagia periodically and suggest adaptations that will improve swallowing and minimize choking. Eating slowly, avoiding distractions during mealtime, adjusting food textures and using adaptive equipment are all helpful in reducing choking. Family members should be taught the Heimlich maneuver.

Most people with HD can be maintained on oral feeding throughout the course of the disease. In later stages, the loss of coordination of oral and pharyngeal muscles will require slow, careful feeding of pureed foods, and beverages will need to be thickened with Thick-It® or related agents to reduce choking. Nutritional needs can be met by liquid supplements alone for some individuals. In some cases, swallowing is so impaired that people with HD suffer hunger, thirst and severe unwanted weight loss. Gastrostomy tubes placed by percutaneous endoscopy or interventional radiology can provide palliation of suffering and afford maintenance of hydration and nutrition in late-stage disease. A discussion around the issue of tube feeding should be held while the individual is still able to express his or her wishes either informally or in an Advance Directive.

Incontinence

Bladder and bowel incontinence may occur in mid to late stage HD. Urinary frequency and urgency are common, and mobility issues can contribute to incontinence. Cognitive impairment and loss of executive function may result in lack of recognition of bladder or rectal fullness, and apathy may prevent timely travel to the commode. Some individuals complain of the frequent urge to urinate or defecate. Urinary retention may occur, and urodynamic testing may reveal a neurogenic bladder. People with HD also frequently suffer from urinary tract infections due to incomplete emptying of the bladder. Setting up a regular schedule for toileting is often helpful. If problems persist or are severe, referral to an urologist or urogynecologist is strongly recommended, as both pharmacologic and behavioral techniques can help significantly.

Seizures

Epileptic seizures occasionally occur in HD. The incidence is around 25% in Juvenile onset HD, and seizures are more likely to occur in younger adults with HD. Other movement disorders such as myoclonus, tics, tremor or dystonia can be mistaken for seizures. Careful history and medical work-up is indicated, together with brain imaging and EEG. If unprovoked seizures are suspected, pharmacologic treatment should be instituted based on the seizure type and concomitant medications.

Weight Loss

Weight loss is common in moderate to late stage HD. The causes are many. Research suggests that metabolic rates are higher in people with HD. Chorea and dystonia require considerable energy and increase the individual's caloric needs. Cognitive decline, behavioral changes, and apathy may make it more difficult to plan, purchase and prepare food. Distractions can interfere with the ability to concentrate on eating, and swallow dysfunction may result in mealtimes that stretch to nearly an hour. Even with the best of care, individuals with marked chorea often lose weight.

Fortunately, most people with HD maintain a high interest in food. Caregivers should be encouraged to prepare food for the person with HD, provide reminders about eating, and offer frequent snacks. Smaller, more frequent meals may reduce stress and improve nutrition. As the disease progresses, assistance with feeding will be required.

Referral to a speech-language pathologist is recommended for a formal swallowing evaluation, once feeding or swallowing difficulties arise. The speech-language pathologist can instruct people with HD and caregivers in techniques to reduce choking, such as changing food textures. Re-consultation with the speech-language pathologist is recommended as difficulties progress. A dietitian or nutritionist may be helpful in developing high calorie dietary plans that promote maintenance of weight and nourishment. If dysphagia is severe, high-protein liquid food supplements should be offered. For a discussion of issues related to the placement of feeding tubes, please see Chapter 8, under *Oral-Motor Dysfunction.*

Conclusions

While motor and neurological impairments in HD are progressive and disabling, currently available treatments will help people with HD and their caregivers with symptomatic management. Strategies that help with difficult behaviors will also benefit movement-related symptoms. Recognition and diagnosis of specific motor and neurological disorders will determine the best therapy. Adaptive equipment, pharmacologic treatment, and multidisciplinary team care, including early referral to allied health specialists will benefit people with HD and their caregivers, optimize functional abilities, and provide relief from symptoms. Effective palliative measures in late stage HD address rigidity and immobility, maintenance of nutrition, relief of pain, and may provide spiritual comfort.

Pain and Pain Management in HD

People with HD often under-report pain, sometimes even in the face of significant obvious injury from trauma or co-morbid illness. This phenomenon can be explained by "unawareness" due to impaired frontal-striatal connections (see Chapter 5). The individual's failure to report pain can make the recognition of serious injury or illness more challenging for caregivers and health professionals. Physicians should be careful not to attribute all medical symptoms to HD alone. Common painful conditions that arise in HD include severe chorea, dystonia, occult fractures and sprains, pressure sores, urinary retention and severe constipation.

In late stage HD, severe muscle rigidity, contractures, chorea, and immobility can all cause pain. The person with HD may not complain of pain on questioning, or communication may be so impaired as to prevent accurate assessment. The physician should look for behavioral changes that may signal pain, including restlessness, screaming, agitation, irritability and anger, resistance to care, or sometimes apathy and withdrawal. Physicians and health professionals should be attentive to conditions that are known to cause pain so that they can offer adequate pain management treatment.

The management of pain in HD may include treatment of chorea, dystonia and rigidity, prevention of injury with fall prevention strategies, protective padding and frequent repositioning, as well as careful attention to urination and bowel regimens to avoid constipation. Some people in early stage HD complain of significant muscle aching or pain. Treatment includes simple analgesics such as acetaminophen or non-steroidal anti-inflammatory (NSAID) drugs. If they fail to help, gabapentin can be quite effective. Pain from tissue and joint injuries should be treated with analgesics.

All people in late stage HD should receive regularly scheduled pain medications to treat the pain of rigidity and immobility. First-line treatment is with acetaminophen or NSAID drugs every 6-8 hours. As later stage immobility progresses, analgesics should be increased in combination with low-dose opiates such as hydrocodone with acetaminophen, and in time, more long-lasting oral or transdermal opiates may be indicated. The addition of opiate therapy requires more aggressive bowel regimens.

Case Study: #1

Treating Chorea

A 44 year old man with a five year history of Huntington's Disease is seen for management of chorea. His symptoms of chorea have gradually increased, and are now constant, affecting his face, trunk and limbs. He complains of clumsiness, often drops items or spills liquids, and has had a few falls. The movements interfere with falling asleep, and his wife complains that he's extremely restless at nighttime. He has had mild cognitive changes due to HD, but no behavioral difficulties. He experienced moderate depression at the time of his diagnosis, but the depression has been well-managed and is stable through treatment with an SSRI. His examination shows mild facial movements, motor impersistence of tongue protrusion, and frequent, moderate-amplitude repetitive irregular movements of his hands. His gait is characterized by frequent lurching movements of the trunk, with brief jerks of his lower legs affecting balance.

He is started on a dose of 12.5 mg q day of tetrabenazine, which is gradually increased to 25 mg BID, with notable improvement in his chorea at follow-up one month later. However, when he returns after three months, his family reports that he's been more withdrawn for the last few weeks, and he admits to feelings of depression and hopelessness. He denies suicidal ideation. His examination reveals slight loss of facial expressivity and psychomotor slowing. He has slight chorea in his limbs and trunk.

The doctor, knowing that a reduction in dosage is often effective for managing depression induced by tetrabenazine, reduces the man's dose to 12.5 mg tid. The man's symptoms of depression improve within a week, and he maintains effective chorea reduction.

Case Study: #2

Treating Chorea

A 58 year old retired teacher with a four year history of HD, with predominant motor symptoms, has significant chorea. She complains that her movements interfere with writing, eating and dressing, and she has tripped and fallen several times. Her chorea is worse at night and significantly interferes with sleep. She has never experienced psychiatric or behavioral difficulties associated with HD. Her examination reveals mild facial chorea and moderate trunkal and limb chorea.

She is started on tetrabenazine, 12.5 mg daily, and the dose is slowly titrated up to 50 mg/day. She returns in 6 weeks, and both she and her spouse report marked improvement in her chorea and insomnia. No side effects have emerged. Her examination confirms the improvement.

Three months later the woman's spouse calls with a report that the woman has developed marked anxiety. She recently saw her primary care physician and was diagnosed as having panic attacks. The doctor recommends reducing the tetrabenazine to 25 mg/day. Three days later the woman is still severely anxious, and the doctor recommends that the medication be stopped.

When the woman returns to the office a week later, her anxiety has resolved, but her chorea has rapidly returned and her insomnia is problematic. A neuroleptic is prescribed on an off-label basis for treatment of chorea. Olanzapine is initiated at a dose of 1.25 mg at bedtime, and the dose is slowly titrated up to 7.5 mg at bedtime. At follow-up two months later, she has gained 9 pounds. Her chorea is significantly improved, her mood is stable, and she is sleeping well. She's advised to take steps to reduce further weight gain and schedule regular monitoring of lipids, and she is maintained on this treatment.

Chapter 5

The Cognitive Disorder

Jane Paulsen, Ph.D.

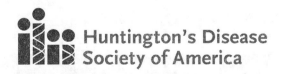

Huntington's Disease
Society of America

The Cognitive Disorder

The cognitive disorder in Huntington's Disease (HD) encompasses a broad variety of cognitive skills, including learning and memory, perceptual skills, executive efficiency and language. The impairments in HD are quite distinct from the highly prevalent dementia associated with Alzheimer's disease, lacking features such as aphasia, amnesia, or agnosia.

This chapter provides an overview of cognitive impairments and the related behavior problems that typically accompany HD. In addition, compensation and adaptation strategies are provided, which physicians may recommend to people with HD, families and other professionals.

Consequences of the Cognitive Disorder

The learning and memory problems associated with HD begin very early in the progression of the disease. There is no evidence that any cognitive dysfunction is evident from birth, but research findings suggest that subclinical cognitive changes can occur 15 years prior to a diagnosis of the movement disorder.

Although currently the clinical diagnosis of HD is based on the presence of the movement disorder, research data and personal stories suggest that the cognitive and behavioral changes are the most debilitating aspect of the disease and place the greatest burden on people with HD and their families.

Even very early in the course of HD, cognitive and behavioral impairments are greater sources of impaired functioning than the movement disorder, both in the work place and at home. In addition, family members report that placement outside the home is more often initiated because of cognitive and behavioral deterioration rather than motor symptoms.

Learning and Memory

Memory problems are a frequently reported symptom of HD. Individuals with the disease have difficulty learning new information and retrieving previously learned information. This appears to be due to a slowed speed of processing and an impaired ability to organize information.

Interestingly, several studies have found that people with HD can demonstrate normal memory if offered in a recognition format, which means that they have stored the information, but have difficulty accessing it at normal speeds. For example: if, rather than asking "can you tell me what time your doctor's appointment is today?," one inquires "is your doctor's appointment at 10:00 or 11:00 today?," people with HD can often answer correctly. Similarly, if people with HD are given a long list of words to learn and are then required to say the words back freely, they perform poorly. But if they are given a list of words and asked to recognize which ones were on the earlier list, they demonstrate good memory.

Explicit vs. Implicit Memory Impairments

The cognitive disorder in HD is distinct from that of other diseases, such as Alzheimer's, in that it affects implicit memories – those collections of coordinated movements and skills that allow an individual to ride a bike, play a musical instrument and perform tasks such as driving a car. Impairment in this area affects even the ability to chew and swallow without choking.

Conditions associated with severe amnesia, such as Korsakoff's syndrome, herpes encephalitis, or Alzheimer's disease, often lead to defective explicit memory, such as recollection of names and dates, while retaining implicit, or unconscious memory, such as the ability to tie one's shoes.

In contrast, older memories of names and dates are often unaffected in people with HD, even as they develop impairments in implicit, or unconscious, motor memory which is essential to driving, playing a musical instrument, or riding a bike. Impairment of unconscious motor memory makes the individual more reliant on conscious memory systems to perform tasks such as driving a car. For the person with HD, skills such as driving will require immense concentration, resulting in increased fatigue, errors, and irritability.

Perceptual Problems

The basic ability to perceive information is often affected very early in HD. The PREDICT-HD observational study has shown perceptual problems arising 8-15 years prior to the movement disorder. Perceptual problems in the prodrome of HD include impairments in emotional recognition, perception of time, smell identification, spatial perception and unawareness.

Symptoms of perceptual problems may not be easily evident in office visits, although they may interfere significantly with the individual's home and work life. Reporting from family and caregivers may be the way that the physician becomes aware of these impairments.

Emotional Recognition

The earliest cognitive impairment detected in a person at-risk for HD is in the ability to recognize emotions. People in the prodrome of HD begin to inaccurately identify which emotion is being communicated in a facial expression. When at-risk individuals were asked to identify whether a facial expression represented fear, sadness, or happiness, performances were significantly impaired. It is hypothesized that this early impairment may be associated with growing difficulties in social relations. It is important to note that understanding of emotions and memory for emotions is intact, it is the identification of emotion based on the complex processing of the face that becomes difficult.

Perception of Time

Research has suggested that people with HD have difficulty with the estimation of time even 8-15 years before motor diagnosis. Spouses often complain that their once-punctual spouse is often late and mis-estimates how long activities will take. When people in the HD prodrome were asked to keep a metronome going after the cued tapping was discontinued, their internal "clock" or timer was inconsistent.

Strategies to Share with Caregivers
To Aid the Person with HD in Time Perception

- *Use frequent, gentle reminders to keep on schedule.*
- *Allow extra time for each task.*
- *Avoid time pressure when possible.*

Spatial Perception

The mental manipulation of personal space becomes impaired as HD progresses. For instance, the judgment of where the body is in relation to walls, corners or tables may be disturbed, resulting in falls and accidents.

Strategies to Share with Caregivers
To Aid the Person with HD in Spatial Perception

- *Keep clear pathways through rooms.*
- *Consider carpeting the floor.*
- *Pad furniture with sharp corners.*

Smell Identification

People in the prodrome of HD performed in the impaired range on a test of smell identification. Although they were able to detect the smells, they were less able to identify what the smell was. Performances on traditional memory tests were intact although smell identification was impaired. The olfactory system appears to be impacted early in the progression of HD.

Unawareness

Awareness of one's own actions and feelings appears to be impaired in at least one-third of people with HD. Although not universal, this perceptual impairment can be associated with significant problems in daily life. Behavior problems reported by family members are often due to impaired perception and unawareness of changes due to HD, which can lead to challenges in providing care.

Unawareness in HD is different from denial, which is commonly described as a psychological inability to cope with distressing circumstances, such as the loss of a loved one, a terminal disease, or a serious injury. In comparison to denial, people with HD often suffer from a lack of insight or self awareness. They may be unable to recognize their own disabilities or evaluate their own behavior.

Unawareness often plays a significant role in seemingly irrational behavior. At first unawareness may be beneficial because it prevents demoralization. However, unawareness may lead to anger and frustration when the individual cannot understand why he can no longer work at the same job, or enjoy the same freedom as before. The HD person with unawareness sometimes feels that people are unjustifiably keeping him away from favored activities such as driving, working, or caring for children, and may attempt to do these things against the advice of family and friends. This type of unawareness can become dangerous.

It is important to distinguish unawareness in HD from the more familiar kind of denial in order to avoid thinking of people with HD as suffering from a purely psychological problem. Unawareness in HD is thought to result from a disruption of the pathways between the frontal regions and the basal ganglia. It is sometimes called "organic denial," or anosognosia, and is a condition that may last a lifetime.

Organic denial can be confusing to health professionals, friends, and family members who may interpret the individual's unawareness of symptoms as a willful decision to ignore what is known to be true, when the reality is that the individual simply does not perceive that what is happening to him or her represents symptoms of a disease.

It may be that the person can talk about problems she is having, such as memory problems, involuntary movements or issues with balance, but not acknowledge that he or she has HD. In such a case, the focus should be on mitigating the individual symptoms without repeatedly confronting the issue of the underlying diagnosis.

Where there is noncompliance with therapy or nursing care because of unawareness, it may be useful to develop a contract that creates incentives for compliance while sidestepping discussion of the diagnosis.

Strategies to Share with Caregivers
To Aid the Person with HD in Addressing Unawareness

- *Allow the person with HD to talk about problems and challenges without having to acknowledge the disease.*
- *Understand that insight in the person with HD may not be an achievable goal.*
- *Counseling may help someone with HD come to terms with limitations that are a result of the diagnosis, without demanding specific insight.*
- *Keep the focus on achieving compliance with behavioral goals, using incentives and even written contracts, if needed.*
- *Accept that the person with HD may never come to "accept" the disease.*

Executive Efficiency

Executive functions involve the highest forms of cognitive processing. Executive processes are universally and significantly impacted in HD. Executive functions involve fundamental abilities that regulate the primary cognitive processes in the brain. These fundamental abilities include (but are not limited to) speed of cognitive processing, attention, planning and organization, initiation, perseveration, impulse control, and other regulatory processes impacting cognition. Changes to cognition are part of a constellation of behavioral and personality changes that are referred to as the "dysexecutive syndrome" in Chapter 6, the Psychiatric Disorder, later in this book.

Speed of Cognitive Processing

One of the earliest and most sensitive indicators of the early signs of HD is a change to the speed of thinking skills. The person at-risk for HD will begin to notice that completion of ordinary mental tasks is more tiring and that more time is required to achieve the same outcome.

It appears that the brain compensates for dysfunctional circuitry by using "effortful" processing to do tasks that were once automatic, and by recruiting alternate areas of the brain for cognitive tasks, all of which slows processing speed.

Attention

A person with HD may complain that he can't "pay attention" as well as he used to. The problem seems to arise during sustained or complex types of attention. Most people with HD will experience difficulty with what is called "divided attention," or the capacity to do two things at once. Divided attention is needed to drive a car while listening to the radio, talking to other passengers or reading a map. For most people, divided attention is impaired when we are tired, sick, or stressed. In HD, divided attention is compromised most of the time.

Strategies to Share with Caregivers
To Aid the Person with HD in Addressing Divided Attention

- *Help the person with HD to do only one thing at a time.*
- *Reduce distractions to the person with HD by turning off radios, television, and telephones when trying to complete a task.*

Planning and Organization

Many people in early stage HD complain of problems with organization and report that they just "can't get things done." They may experience difficulties in planning, organization, sequencing and prioritizing which affect their ability to fulfill responsibilities at home and at work. All of these are executive functions that are affected by the changes in the brain caused by HD.

Daily tasks, such as attempts to follow a recipe, to maintain a daily planner, to complete a list of household errands, or to fill out applications or forms may become difficult and frustrating, leading to outbursts of irritation and emotion.

Strategies to Share with Caregivers
To Aid the Person with HD in Planning and Organization

- *Provide the HD person with consistent schedules and routines to help compensate for problems with organization.*
- *Maintain a highly structured environment for the HD person where each day is basically the same.*
- *Establish a central location for posting a daily schedule with lists and tasks to be accomplished each day for the person with HD. Even those who never before used daily planners or computer calendars may need to start.*
- *Rely on routines which can be easier for the person with HD to initiate or continue without guidance.*
- *Make lists which help organize tasks needed for a person with HD to do an activity.*
- *Prompt each step of an activity with external cues (routines, lists, familiar verbal cues) for the person with HD.*
- *Offer limited choices to the person with HD and avoid open ended questions.*
- *Use short sentences with the HD person that contain just 1-2 pieces of information.*

Lack of Initiation

Some family members complain that the person with HD "just sits around all day and won't do anything." Regulation of behavior involves getting started, maintaining the desired behavior, and stopping unwanted behaviors. The initiation, or starting of an activity, conversation or behavior is often compromised in HD. A lack of initiation is often misinterpreted as laziness, apathy or lack of interest, and may be a reason for poor performance at work.

Once started, the person with HD may be able to execute the behaviors adequately (i.e. compute taxes, calculate sales, administrate employees, teach school), but may be unable to organize and initiate the behaviors at the appropriate time. External initiation often helps the person with HD remain active and able to participate in both social and work activities. Keeping a daily routine can minimize the need for internal initiation.

Perseveration

Spouses often report that the person with HD becomes behaviorally rigid, and tends to get stuck on an idea or task. Perseveration, or being fixed on a specific thought or action, can occur when behaviors are inadequately regulated by the brain.

Established routines can help avoid problems. An activity that is atypical for the established routine may be challenging for the person with HD. For instance, travel out of town, or a visit to the doctor or dentist, may disrupt a safe routine. Caregivers can help the person with HD prepare for new or unusual events with gentle reminders. If anxiety is an issue, caregivers should tell the person with HD only a day or a few hours before the event.

Impulsivity

Some degree of impulsivity and dysregulation of behaviors is quite common in HD. Over time, HD will cause difficulties with impulse control and problem behaviors, such as irritability, temper outbursts, acting without thinking, and inappropriate sexual behavior.

Strategies to Share with Caregivers
To Aid the Person with HD in Reducing Impulsivity

- *Since the person with HD cannot control their responses, a predictable daily schedule can reduce confusion, fear and, as a result, outbursts.*
- *It is possible that a behavior by the person with HD is a reasonable response to something that needs attention. Caregivers must not be too quick to discount it as an outburst.*
- *It is important for caregivers to remain calm. Staying calm may help the person with HD to calm down and will allow the caregiver to think and not react emotionally and impulsively.*
- *It is important to let the person with HD know that yelling is not the best way to get attention and offer alternative methods.*
- *Although hurtful and embarrassing things are being said, in general, the person with HD is not doing this intentionally. Caregivers should be reassured that it is often the HD that is talking.*

- The person with HD may be remorseful after an outburst. Caregivers can be sensitive to efforts to apologize and not badger the person with HD after the fact. It won't help, as the lack of control is likely not by choice.

- Medications may be helpful for outbursts and sexually inappropriate behavior. Physicians should talk with caregivers about these options.

Irritability and Temper Outbursts

Among the most common complaints from HD families are irritability and temper outbursts. As symptoms of the cognitive disorder, these outbursts may be caused by the loss of impulse control, from confusion or feelings of being overwhelmed, from a disruption in the ability to track time, or by frustration that one's needs (however reasonable or unreasonable) are not being met. Irritability can also occur due to an unawareness of thirst or hunger, which is a common symptom of HD.

Irritability may also be a symptom of depression. Assessing for and treating a mood disorder may diminish irritability and temper outbursts. However, irritability or outbursts are a common symptom of HD, even in the absence of a mood disorder.

Identifying the underlying causes of irritability and temper outbursts may help diminish their frequency and severity. Frustration plays a major role in triggering outbursts. People with HD are continually challenged by previously routine tasks or activities that they now experience as overwhelming. HD results in a progressive loss of abilities that often "sneak up." People with HD have confided that "I didn't realize I could no longer do it."

The physician may or may not experience an outburst during a normal office visit. Caregiver reporting may be an important means of tracking outbursts and their severity. In some instances, the person with HD will recover from the temper outburst quite quickly and forget all about it, leaving the family shaken and disturbed. You may find that family members or caregivers wish to speak with you privately about their loved one's irritability and emotional outbursts.

While irritability often passes quickly, outbursts do have the potential to become violent. Safety should always come first and caregivers should be encouraged to prepare an exit strategy for leaving the house or calling for help if an outburst threatens to get out of control.

Treatment for irritability and temper outbursts are discussed in detail in Chapter 6, the Psychiatric Disorder, later in this book.

Strategies to Share with Caregivers
To Aid the Person with HD in Reducing Irritability and Outbursts

- Caregivers should learn the signals, verbal or nonverbal, that the individual is frustrated or upset.

- Attempts should be made to anticipate situations which trigger frustration and either avoid them or provide diversions.

- The environment should be kept as calm and controlled as possible.

- Caregivers should be encouraged to talk to the physician about their personal frustrations with the loved one's limitations.

- *Stay calm and speak quietly.*
- *Avoid confrontations and ultimatums.*
- *Sit down and limit hand gestures.*
- *Redirect the HD person away from the source of anger.*
- *Acknowledge the individual's irritability as a symptom of frustration.*
- *Try not to take cruel words personally.*
- *Leave the area if the outburst threatens to become violent.*

Language

Communication, or the transfer of information from one person to another, requires a complex integration of thought, muscle control, and breathing. HD can impair all three of these functions. The most prominent language difficulties in people with HD are (1) speaking clearly (articulation), (2) starting conversation (initiation), and (3) organizing what's coming in and what's going out (cognitive processing). Misarticulation is discussed in Chapter 4, the Motor Dysfunction.

Impaired Initiation of Speech

Due to changes in the speed of cognitive processing, word finding is often impaired in HD, although the knowledge of vocabulary is retained. In addition to speed limitations, the brain fails to regulate the sequence and amount of traveling information, resulting in impairments in starting and stopping.

Disorganization of Language Content

In contrast to the basic impairments in language output, the basic capacity to understand language remains relatively intact in HD. Even in later stages of the disease, language comprehension may remain when the ability to speak is significantly diminished. This fact is important to communicate to family members, staff at care facilities and other healthcare professionals. Even if a person with HD cannot express herself, it is likely that she can understand what is being said.

Difficulties with word usage are rare in people with HD, as are frank aphasia or impairments in semantic memory. The trouble that occurs in people with HD is an inability to organize the outgoing and incoming language, resulting in miscommunication.

Strategies to Share with Caregivers
To Aid the Person with HD in Improving Communication

- *Allow additional time for the person with HD to respond to questions.*
- *Try yes or no questions to speed a response from a person with HD.*
- *Use short simple sentences and assess understanding frequently.*
- *Know that even if the person with HD cannot speak, they can understand what is being said.*

Functional Correlates of Cognitive Impairments

Typically, the first impairment in functional activity is losing the ability to work in accustomed employment. Most often people with early symptoms can continue to remain gainfully employed but will change jobs or move to a position that might be less demanding. Some people with HD have been able to remain employed for a significant amount of time after symptoms begin. Maintenance of employment requires that the person be flexible and willing to consider other levels of paid activity. The majority of people (88%) maintain employment until after a motor diagnosis of HD is given. The best indicators of being able to maintain an accustomed job, without a job change, are better performances on a task of psychomotor speed, fewer motor signs, and higher energy (less fatigue).

The decision to retire or apply for disability is an important one that should be considered with input from occupational therapists, social workers, psychologists and physicians. There is no "one size fits all" with regard to becoming eligible for disability. Cognitive performances can be used to help counsel what jobs might be most readily completed with the least amount of stress, and the current family financial situation, as well as the activity and participation needs of the individual, must be considered.

The Progression of Cognitive Impairments: Prodrome through Late Stage

Even in the prodrome of HD some individuals experience mild forms of cognitive impairment. In people most near to receiving a motor diagnosis of HD, about 73% are performing at least one and a half standard deviations below their peers. The most common reason for the early cognitive issues in HD is slowed processing speed. Nevertheless, many people with HD can continue to function at normal levels if they can allow themselves extra time to complete tasks. A modification of schedules and expectations is essential to maintain the highest levels of activity and performance, and to avoid depressed moods due to failures.

Although performance in IQ tests often remains within the normal range in the early stages of the disease, deficits are evident in speed of processing, cognitive flexibility (or the ability to shift topics readily), and the organization of complex information. The most sensitive indicator of early HD on the Mini-Mental State Examination is serial sevens (the ability to subtract 7 from 100 serially) and the most sensitive subscale on the Mattis Dementia Rating Scale is initiation (the ability to begin and maintain verbal and motor behaviors).

Longitudinal studies of the cognitive decline in HD have suggested that speed, organization, and initiation of behavior are impaired in early HD, constructional impairments worsen in mid stage HD, and some abilities remain relatively spared (memory, language comprehension) even in the later stages of the disease. Clinically, as the disease progresses, the severity of cognitive impairments increases and individuals are often unable to speak or communicate their views in late stages. It is likely that most people with HD continue to understand and remember even after their ability to communicate their views and opinions declines. For this reason an early discussion of communication devices, such as computerized speech production or letter board, or simple hand gestures, is essential.

Summary

Several studies, such as PREDICT-HD, have suggested that cognitive impairments are a significant source of impaired functioning in HD and often create a greater burden for HD families than the movement disorder.

The cognitive disorder in HD affects "implicit memory" – the unconscious memory of how to play a musical instrument, drive a car, even chew and swallow without choking. These memory problems, combined with the disruption to executive functioning and slowed mental processing caused by the disease, force the individual to rely on conscious memory systems to perform ordinary tasks, requiring immense concentration and causing fatigue, frustration and irritability.

The cognitive disorder also manifests during the prodrome of the disease as impairments in emotional recognition, perception of time, smell identification, spatial perception and unawareness of symptoms.

In recent years, research has shown that the impact of HD on cognition and behavior may appear a decade or more before the movement disorder. The physician must be alert to changes in cognitive and executive processes, in order to help the individual and their family adopt adaptive strategies early on, so that the person with HD can maintain optimal functioning at home and at work. Cognitive problems may not be easily evident in typical office visits. The physician should be alert for reports from caregivers about early changes to the speed and quality of thought and perception.

Cognitive Assessment: the Unified Huntington's Disease Rating Scale (UHDRS)

The most highly used tool to assess HD is the Unified Huntington's Disease Rating Scale (UHDRS). It is a standardized measure used in assessing the progression of HD.

The components of the UHDRS are:

- *Motor Assessment*
- *Cognitive Assessment*
- *Behavioral Assessment*
- *Independence Scale*
- *Functional Assessment*
- *Total Functional Capacity (TFC)*

In addition, the UHDRS examines medical history, family history, and medications.

To measure cognition, The UHDRS uses three tasks:

1) Symbol Digit Modalities test: which requires the person to match as many symbols and numbers as quickly as possible in 90 seconds;

2) Stroop Color Word test: which requires the person to name the colors of boxes, read words and name the colors of ink in a word. Each task is allowed 45 seconds and the score is the number of items correctly read aloud.

3) Verbal Fluency test: which requires the person to say aloud as many words that begin with a specified letter in 60 seconds.

These three tasks do not begin to cover the numerous aspects of cognition that are impaired by HD. The tasks do, however, provide a valid estimate of performance on one of the most sensitive indicators of cognition in HD: speed of processing. Physicians wishing to obtain a copy of the complete UHDRS should visit the Huntington Study Group website at www.huntington-study-group.org and click on the Resources tab.

Case Study: #1

The Cognitive Disorder: The Impact of Knowing

A 50 year old male with no noticeable chorea is still working as a bank executive but presents to the HD Center due to increased irritability and depressed mood. An antidepressant is prescribed and a neuropsychological evaluation is requested. Findings reveal that intellect is in the superior range but learning and speed are in the average range. Neuropsychological feedback is given as well as strategies for compensation for supposed cognitive declines.

One month later the man reports that he was able to modify his work schedule and duties to maximize his efforts and decrease his stress. His depression and irritability decreased and he was able to continue working.

Case Study: #2

The Cognitive Disorder: Initiation

A 60 year old mother, living with her daughter, reported that her learning, memory and language were good, her mood great, and her interest in activities high. She enjoyed and cared about many things in her life but was disappointed that she "never did anything anymore." Both she and her family reported that her once-active lifestyle had changed to "sitting around all day watching TV." After complaining about her inactivity to others, including her family, it was agreed that the family would try to be the "frontal lobe" and help her with activities.

This strategy worked very well. She was a good follower and enjoyed the activities that friends and family encouraged her to attend or participate in. However, after about six weeks, it became evident that the family was experiencing significant distress and fatigue in having to guide and begin activities. The family was small and all of the family members had full-time commitments to work and/or school. They grew tired of providing constant initiation for their mother/grandmother and began to neglect her. One day, her daughter came home with an abandoned puppy. At the family's request, the mother adopted the puppy. The next time she and her family were seen in support group, the whole family announced that the puppy had become the mother's "starter switch" and now initiated much of the activity for the mother. The puppy initiated playtime, dinnertime, time to go outside to the bathroom and time to go for a walk. The mother was no longer inactive and her quality of life was significantly improved for everyone (thankfully, the puppy house-trained quickly!).

Chapter 6

The Psychiatric
Disorder

Adam Rosenblatt, M.D.

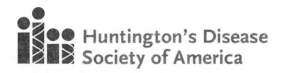 **Huntington's Disease
Society of America**

The Psychiatric Disorder

Psychiatric symptoms have long been understood to be a common and inherent part of Huntington's Disease (HD). In the classic description of the condition which bears his name, George Huntington referred to "the tendency to insanity, and sometimes that form of insanity which leads to suicide…" Most physicians understand this in the abstract, yet people with HD with psychiatric problems suffer from under-diagnosis and under-treatment. This is regrettable, because psychiatric problems in HD are often the most disabling and yet the most treatable.

Psychiatric problems in HD tend to fall into three categories. The first consists of mental illnesses which are common in the general population and are readily recognized by physicians, especially major depression, which has been estimated to affect 40% of people with HD at some point during their illness. Other frequently encountered syndromes may include mania, obsessive compulsive disorder, and various delusional and psychotic disorders.

The second category consists of psychiatric problems which are not often found in the general population but are common in neuropsychiatric patients, particularly those with injuries and diseases affecting the sub-cortical areas of the brain or the frontal lobes, such as HD, strokes, Parkinson's disease, head injuries and various forms of dementia. This usually takes the form of a constellation of behavioral and personality changes which can include apathy, irritability, disinhibition, perseveration, jocularity, obsessiveness, and impaired judgment. These changes are collectively described by various names including *organic personality syndrome, frontal lobe syndrome*, or *dysexecutive syndrome*, which will be the term used here. These changes are not always severe or obvious enough to be apparent to physicians during regular office visits, but the syndrome is so common in HD as to be virtually universal.

Finally there are those psychiatric issues, such as delirium, "agitation," or sexual disorders, which are difficult to characterize, perhaps because they depend so heavily on the interaction between the person with HD, the disease, and the environment.

This chapter will address the major psychiatric manifestations of HD and their treatment, including some illustrative case vignettes, and will also include a discussion of the standard diagnostic codes which may be used for billing and insurance purposes.

Psychiatric Syndromes Common in the General Population

Depression

It has been estimated that the lifetime prevalence of major depression in people with HD is about 40%. However, most people with HD do not experience depression and are able to adapt gradually to having HD and the losses it entails. They may become demoralized at various times but do not develop a clinical syndrome. Most researchers believe that syndromic depression in HD should be looked at as a direct neurological symptom of the brain disease.

Signs and Symptoms of Depression

- *Depressed or irritable mood*

- *Loss of interest or pleasure in activities*

- *Change in appetite or weight loss*

- *Insomnia or hypersomnia*

- *Loss of energy*

- *Feelings of worthlessness or guilt*

- *Impaired concentration*

- *Thoughts of death or suicide*

- *Loss of libido*

- *Feelings of hopelessness*

- *Social withdrawal*

- *Psychomotor retardation or agitation*

(Based on DSM-IV criteria)

Physicians and family members must resist the temptation to interpret an individual's depressed mood or suicidal thoughts as an appropriate reaction to having a fatal neurodegenerative disease, not requiring treatment. People with HD who have a depressive syndrome, even when there appear to be environmental triggers, usually respond to standard treatments, including medications and psychotherapy. Because depression in HD appears directly related to the brain disease, and cognitive impairment may limit the individual's ability to participate in counseling, pharmacotherapy is usually indicated.

Major depression in someone with HD is not "understandable" and suicide is not "appropriate." A suicidal person with HD has treatable major depression until proven otherwise.

Diagnosing Major Depression

Major depression is a clinical syndrome, recognizable by a constellation of signs and symptoms. Use of diagnostic criteria helps to distinguish major depression from demoralization, bereavement, and other symptoms common in HD, such as weight loss, poor concentration, or apathy. Individuals with major depression have a sustained low mood, often accompanied by changes in self-attitude, such as feelings of worthlessness or guilt, a loss of interest or pleasure in activities, changes in appetite and sleep, particularly early morning awakening, loss of energy, and hopelessness. Depressed individuals often feel worse in the morning than in the afternoon.

In severe cases of depression, individuals may have delusions or hallucinations, which tend to match their depressed mood. A person with HD may hear voices berating him or urging him to commit suicide, or may have the delusion that he will be going to jail, or that he has killed his family. Depressed individuals often display psychomotor retardation, a slowing of speech and movement, as a result of depression. In extreme cases they can appear stuporous or catatonic.

In some cases of depression, the presenting complaint may be something other than a low mood. For example a depressed person may complain initially of insomnia, anxiety, or pain. It is vital to get the whole story, because symptomatic treatment for any of these complaints, e.g. sleeping pills, tranquilizers, or narcotics, could be worse than no treatment at all. Even in the absence of a specific complaint of depressed mood, a physician may decide to treat depression presumptively if the person has the other symptoms. People with HD sometimes have trouble identifying or describing their emotional state. Depression in such an individual could be suggested by changes in sleep or appetite, agitation, tearfulness, or rapid functional decline. In such circumstances the diagnosis of depression should be considered.

In evaluating a person with HD with depression, the physician also needs to consider other secondary causes. The individual's medical history should be reviewed for conditions such as hypothyroidism, stroke, head injury or exposure to certain drugs associated with mood changes, such as steroids, tetrabenazine, or excessive alcohol.

Pharmacotherapy for Depression

There is no single preferred antidepressant for treating depression in HD. The treating physician should bear in mind that people with HD are sensitive to the cognitive side effects of some antidepressants and are easily made delirious, as if they were much older than their chronological age. Therefore the older agents such as tricyclic antidepressants and monoamine oxidase inhibitors should generally be avoided, or at least not considered first line. Most physicians would start with a selective serotonin reuptake inhibitor (SSRI), such as fluoxetine (Prozac®), sertraline (Zoloft®), paroxetine (Paxil®), citalopram (Celexa®), or escitalopram (Lexapro®) for reasons of safety and tolerability, and because some experts regard them as particularly helpful for the dysexecutive behavioral symptoms of HD, which are discussed later in this chapter. Most are now available in inexpensive generic formulations. Initial side effects may be GI upset or diarrhea, and increased anxiety or insomnia (although these complaints are sometimes actually aspects of the depression itself, in which case they should eventually respond to the treatment). Other popular choices include buproprion (Wellbutrin®), venlafaxine (Effexor®), duloxetine (Cymbalta®) and desvenelafaxine (Pristiq®). Given the sensitivity of people with HD to side effects, antidepressants should be started at a low dose (such as 25-50 mg of sertraline or 10 mg of escitalopram) and advanced gradually.

The SSRIs, and other antidepressants, are sometimes initially stimulating. On rare occasions, they may galvanize individuals with symptoms of anergic depression (lack of interest, energy or motivation) into sudden self-destructive action. This may underlie the warning, now carried in the U.S. package insert of all antidepressant drugs, that antidepressants may worsen suicidal impulses and behaviors, particularly in adolescents. Most psychiatrists are aware of a person who committed suicide just when his family and friends thought he was beginning to get better. This does not mean that antidepressant drugs should not be used, since the risks of untreated depression are far worse, but that individuals beginning treatment for depression should have a discussion with their physician about suicidal impulses, should be cautioned to report such symptoms, and should enlist their support network of family and friends.

Treating Depression and Psychosis

If the person's depression is accompanied by delusions, hallucinations, or significant agitation, it may be necessary to add an antipsychotic medication to the regimen, preferably in low doses to minimize the risk of sedation, rigidity, or parkinsonism. If the neuroleptic is being used for a purely psychiatric purpose, and not for suppression of chorea, the physician may want to prescribe one of the newer agents such as risperidone (Risperdal®), olanzepine (Zyprexa®), quetiapine (Seroquel®), ziprasidone (Geodon®) or aripiprazole (Abilify®). These drugs may have a lower incidence of side effects and appear to be just as effective. Neuroleptics are sometimes used to augment the effects of antidepressant medications and aripiprazole and quetiapine actually have formal indications for particular instances of depression. Among the older neuroleptics, which are much less expensive, the high potency agents such as haloperidol (Haldol®) or fluphenazine (Prolixin®) tend to be less sedating, but cause more parkinsonism, which is why they have often been used in small doses to suppress chorea. Benzodiazepines, particularly short acting drugs such as lorazepam (Ativan®), may be another good choice for the short-term management of agitation. In any case, neuroleptics and benzodiazepines used for acute agitation should be tapered as soon as the clinical picture allows.

Some Psychiatric Medications Commonly Used in Treating the Psychiatric Symptoms of HD

Note: There is only one medication that is specifically approved by the FDA for use in HD – Tetrabenazine, a chorea treatment. The following medications are suggestions based on the clinical experience of the author. Physicians should carefully review the pharmaceutical manufacturers' materials regarding dosage and potential side effects before prescribing any medication.

Antidepressants
(used for depression and sometimes for irritability and anxiety as well):
SSRIs:
- Sertraline (Zoloft®)   - Paroxetine (Paxil®)
- Citalopram (Celexa®)   - Fluoxetine (Prozac®)
- Escitalopram (Lexapro®)

Others:
- Buproprion (Wellbutrin®)   - Venlafaxine (Effexor®)

Neuroleptics
(used for psychosis and sometimes for irritability or for chorea suppression)
- *Atypical Antipsychotics:*
- Olanzepine (Zyprexa®)   - Ziprasidone (Geodon®)
- Quetiapine (Seroquel®)   - Aripiprazole (Abilify®)

High Potency Antipsychotics (sometimes also used for chorea suppression) :

- Haloperidol (Haldol®)   - Risperidone (Risperdal®)
- Fluphenazine (Prolixin®)

Electroconvulsive therapy (ECT) has also been found effective in depressed people with HD. This treatment should be considered if a person does not respond to several good trials of medication, or if a more immediate intervention is needed for reasons of safety. For example a severely depressed person may be refusing food and fluids, or may be very actively suicidal. ECT may be particularly effective in treating delusional depression.

Depressed individuals should always be asked about substance abuse. Substance abuse, particularly of alcohol, can be both a consequence and a cause of depression, making treatment difficult if not addressed, and significantly increasing the risk of suicide.

Suicide

Suicide is alarmingly common in people with HD, possibly because of the frequent co-morbidity of depression and personality changes resulting in disinhibition and impulsive behavior, but that does not mean that suicide is not preventable.

Depressed individuals should always be asked about suicide, and this should be regularly re-assessed. It is a misconception that suicidal individuals will not admit to these feelings. The question should be asked in a non-intimidating, matter-of-fact way, such as "Have you been feeling so bad that you sometimes think life isn't worth living?" Or, "Have you even thought about suicide?" If the person acknowledges these feelings, the clinician needs to ask more questions to evaluate the severity of the situation and decide on the best course of action. Are the feelings just a passive wish to die or has the person actually thought out a specific suicidal plan? Does the person have the means to commit suicide? Has she prepared for a suicide, such as by loading a gun or hoarding pills? Can the person identify any factors which are preventing her from killing herself? What social supports are present? Some individuals, although having suicidal thoughts, may be at low risk if they have a good relationship with their doctor, have family support, and have no specific plans. Others may be so dangerous to themselves that they require emergency hospitalization.

Although there are instances of non-depressed individuals with HD harboring chronic suicidal feelings, most, if not all, suicidal people with HD are suffering from major depression and can be treated successfully. In cases of completed suicide in HD of which there are first-hand knowledge, the person was usually well understood by his family to be suffering from depression and attempts at treatment had been initiated, but sadly proved insufficient. If the clinician is unsure, the person should be treated presumptively. This is not to say that a person with HD, particularly early in the course of the disease, may not express a fear of becoming helpless one day, or a desire not to live past a certain degree of impairment. A physician should listen supportively to these concerns, realizing that most individuals in this situation will be able to adapt if they are not suffering from depression.

Author's opinion:

It cannot be overstressed that suicide in HD is a preventable manifestation of disease. The concept of a "rational" suicide in someone with HD, a person who dispassionately "chooses" to "take his own life" before symptoms become too advanced, is a myth. Suicide is devastating to the people left behind and increases the risk of suicide in the next generation. It must not be rationalized, romanticized, or accepted.

Case Study: #1

The Psychiatric Disorder: Preventing Suicide

Mr. H, a 59 year old married man with mild Huntington's Disease is seen in a hospital-based clinic for a routine follow-up appointment. His wife mentions that he has not been himself lately. He has been withdrawn, frequently tearful, not showing interest in his previous activities such as gardening and going to yard sales, and talking frequently of "after I'm gone" even though he is expected to live many more years. He seems to be sleeping poorly as she has often awakened to find him out of bed at night.

At his last visit he was prescribed an antidepressant, but he has not been taking it, saying that "It won't help me. Nothing can help me." He also did not call the psychiatrist to whom he was referred. He admits to the doctor that he has been thinking of killing himself and is he convinced that, rather than being harmed by his suicide, his wife and children will be better off without him. The doctor asks him if he has any firearms at home and he replies that his wife and brother have removed his shotguns and rifles, but that he has a pistol that he plans to use to kill himself the following weekend. His plans make perfect sense to him because "There's no cure for HD. I'm not allowed to drive or hunt anymore and I can't support my family."

The doctor takes the man's wife aside and explains that it will be necessary to hospitalize Mr. H because he is suffering from severe depression and is an acute danger to himself. She says that she is relieved, but doubts he will enter the hospital voluntarily. When Mr. H is told that he will need to be admitted, he becomes distraught and lies down on the floor of the examination room. His wife begins crying and asks if there is some other way to treat Mr. H. She is also worried about the cost of a hospital admission and adds that their adult son will be very angry at the treatment of his father.

When a staff member takes Mrs. H into another room for a cup of coffee, the doctor calls for hospital security and three officers remove Mr. H. from the floor, place him on a stretcher, and escort him to the emergency department where he is examined, certified, and admitted to an inpatient psychiatric unit as an involuntary patient.

Mania

While depression is the most common mood disorder in HD, a smaller number of people with HD will become manic, displaying elevated or irritable mood, overactivity, decreased need for sleep, impulsiveness, and grandiosity. Some may alternate between sustained periods of depression and mania, with times of normal mood in between, a condition known as bipolar disorder. It is easy to over-diagnose mania or bipolar disorder in HD because many of the facets of the dysexecutive syndrome of HD (q.v.) such as irritability, impulsivity, or disinhibition can mimic the symptoms. This is an important distinction to make because most of the useful interventions for the dysexecutive syndrome are not pharmacological and many of the drugs used to treat mania are fairly toxic. In genuine mania there should be a sustained elevation of mood, lasting days or weeks, not just periodic impulsive actions or temper flare-ups in response to frustration. Mania is also usually accompanied by "vegetative changes" such as increased appetite, increased energy, and a decreased need for sleep.

People with mania are usually treated with anticonvulsants and neuroleptics. Lithium is still a popular drug for people with idiopathic bipolar disorder, but has not been reported as particularly helpful in people with HD and is rarely used. It also has a narrow therapeutic range, particularly in individuals whose food and fluid intake may be spotty.

Therapy beginning with divalproex sodium (Depakote®) at a low dose such as 125 to 250 mg po bid and gradually increasing to efficacy, or to reach a blood level of 50-150 mcg/ml is recommended. A dose of 500 mg po bid is fairly typical, but some people with HD will require as much as several grams per day. Several other anticonvulsants are sometimes used for treatment of mania, including lamotrigine (Lamictal®), topiramate (Topamax®), and carbamazepine (Tegretol®).

The recommended blood levels for these drugs were established on the basis of their anticonvulsant properties, so it is important to remember that a person with HD may show a good psychiatric response below the minimum "therapeutic" level (but generally should not exceed the maximum level in any case). Divalproex carries a small risk of liver function abnormalities and blood dyscrasias, so LFTs, and CBC should be routinely monitored every few months and clinicians should be alert for suggestive symptoms. Divalproex is also associated with neural tube defects when used during pregnancy.

Manic people with HD, particularly those who are very agitated or who have delusions and hallucinations, may require a neuroleptic, or possibly a benzodiazepine for immediate control of these symptoms. As discussed for depression, the doctor may wish to prescribe one of the newer antipsychotics which have fewer parkinsonian side effects. In cases of extreme agitation, a rapidly acting injectable agent may be necessary.

Obsessions and Compulsions

Obsessions are recurrent, intrusive thoughts or impulses. A compulsion is a repetitive performance of a routine, such as hand washing. Compulsions are sometimes related to obsessions, such as an obsessive concern with germs. Obsessions are usually a source of anxiety and the individual may struggle to put them aside, whereas the acting out of compulsions generally relieves anxiety and may not be as strongly resisted.

The full psychiatric syndrome of Obsessive Compulsive Disorder (OCD) is rare in HD, but people with HD often become preoccupied with a particular idea or routine. These individuals may worry about germs or contamination, or engage in excessive checking of switches or locks. Sometimes people with HD will become fixated on an episode of being wronged in the past (e.g. fired from a job, divorced, driver's license revoked), and then bring it up constantly, or become preoccupied with some perceived need, such as a desire to go shopping, or to eat a certain food.

If obsessions or compulsions interfere with the individual's quality of life, but do not meet the criteria for the full syndrome, serotonergic antidepressants, typically used to treat OCD, may ameliorate the behavior. The use of the tricyclic antidepressant clomipramine (Anafranil®) has largely been superseded by the SSRIs. For relentless perseverative behavior unresponsive to these agents, one might consider neuroleptics.

Delusions and Hallucinations

Chronic psychosis and schizophrenia-like conditions are uncommon in HD. The onset of delusions or hallucinations should prompt a search for specific causes or precipitating factors, including mood disorders, delirium related to metabolic or neurologic derangements, or intoxication with or withdrawal from illicit or prescription drugs. Once these possibilities have been eliminated, neuroleptics may be employed to treat the schizophrenia-like syndromes.

Some individuals may respond completely and others only partly, reporting that "voices" have been reduced to a mumble, or become less preoccupied with delusional concerns. Neuroleptics are also used to control chorea and some very resistant individuals may be convinced to accept an antipsychotic as part of a treatment for the suppression of involuntary movements.

In our experience there is a subset of people with HD whose delusions are extremely tenacious. This may represent the interplay between the delusion itself and the personality changes common in HD. Or perhaps the "delusion" in this case is better thought of as a preoccupation or an over-valued idea. People with delusions will rarely respond to being argued with, but a clinician may certainly express skepticism regarding a delusional belief. Caregivers should be encouraged to respond diplomatically, to appreciate that the delusions are symptoms of a disease, and to avoid direct confrontation if the issue is not crucial.

Case Study: #2

The Psychiatric Disorder: Delusions

A 63 year old divorced woman with HD believes that she is having a love affair with her internist. Her family reports that the man in question was her physician, but that he retired several years ago, is not currently caring for her, and has no idea of the relationship that she believes they share. She insists that he loves her in return and intends to marry her. Her children reminded her that the doctor is already married and she told them that he plans to leave his wife for her.

She tells her psychiatrist that she can hear the internist sending her messages of love at night, because they live on opposite sides of a lake and his voice carries across the water. Her delusions have so far proven unresponsive to three different antipsychotic drugs and usually do not interfere with her daily activities. The current stumbling block, however, is that her family wants her to make the transition to assisted living and she refuses to go, insisting that her gentleman friend will care for her at home.

Psychiatric Problems Specific to HD and other Neuropsychiatric Conditions

The Dysexecutive Syndrome

It has often been said that depression is the most common psychiatric problem in HD. That is not entirely true. While depression may be the most common conventional diagnosis given to people with HD, there is another syndrome - a constellation of behavioral and personality changes - which is so common in HD as to be virtually universal.

These changes are known by a variety of names, including the *dysexecutive syndrome, organic personality syndrome,* or "frontal lobe" syndrome, although this latter is a pseudo-anatomical term, because the frontal lobes are relatively spared in HD, with damage mainly occurring in the subcortical structures which are connected to them.

The dysexecutive syndrome is easy to recognize but somewhat difficult to characterize. It can be easy to under-estimate the impact of the personality changes that make up the syndrome and not give them the clinical attention they deserve. Essentially, there are both disinhibited symptoms such as perseveration (persistent repetition of a word, phrase or gesture), irritability, impulsivity, and jocularity, and deficit symptoms, such as apathy, loss of spontaneity, and indifference. Both kinds of symptoms can co-exist in the same individual. For example, a man with HD may watch the same television station all day, seeming to take little interest in the content, but becomes furious if someone tries to change the channel. Although they may be different sides of the same coin, we will deal with some of the major components of the executive dysfunction syndrome separately, for the purpose of discussing treatment.

Families may have a difficult time dealing with the dysexecutive syndrome. The family may be confronted with someone who looks and sounds just like the wife, sister, friend or mother she used to be, but who shows no interest in previous responsibilities, is capable of callous actions and statements, and who commits grievous errors in judgment despite repeated negative consequences.

It is important to note that a common neurological consequence of HD is unawareness of symptoms. The individual with the disease may not notice the progressive change in their behavior and may dismiss concerns raised by the family. Insight is often an early casualty of the dysexecutive syndrome.

The family should be encouraged to let go of the belief that they can "reason" the individual with HD into more responsible and insightful behavior. Successful management of the dysexecutive syndrome usually consists of maintaining safety, avoiding unnecessary conflict, reducing the number of choices and decisions the person with HD has to make, helping him or her establish a routine, and judicious use of medications. Minimizing stress and conflict in these ways will give the person with HD the best opportunities to be more authentically "himself." More information on management strategies can be found in the "HDSA Family Guide to HD," available on the HDSA website, www.hdsa.org.

Apathy

Apathy is both an emotional and a cognitive syndrome in that the apathetic person lacks emotional investment in his activities and surroundings, but also has difficulty generating new behaviors and initiating activities. Apathy is extremely common in HD and very distressing to caregivers.

Apathetic individuals become unmotivated and uninterested in their surroundings. They lose enthusiasm and lack spontaneity. Performance at work or school becomes sluggish. It can be a source of conflict between individuals and caregivers, who know the person is physically capable of activities but "won't" do them. Apathetic individuals may be uninterested or even resistant to treatment, because, by definition, they do not care, although there have been instances of insightful people with apathy, who request treatment because they are aware of the effects their apathy is having on their families. Families need education and support in this regard. They need to know that their loved one is not bothered by the apathy, and that the family can adopt a combination of exhortation and accommodation to address the condition.

Apathy can be hard to distinguish from depression. Apathetic individuals, like those with depression, may be sluggish, quiet, and disengaged. They may talk slowly, or not at all. By and large apathetic people will say they are not sad, but in distinguishing between the two, it is important to ask not only about the person's mood, but about other depressive symptoms as well, such as a change in sleeping or eating patterns, feelings of guilt, or suicidal thoughts.

Apathy and depression may also co-exist. Depressed people who also suffer from apathy should be treated aggressively for their depression, which may cause the other symptoms to improve. Individuals with primary apathy sometimes respond to psychostimulants such as methylphenidate (Ritalin®), pemoline (Cylert®) or dextroamphetamine (Dexedrine®). These medicines are highly abusable and may exacerbate irritability, so they should be used with caution. It may be more prudent to first make a trial of a non-sedating antidepressant, such as an SSRI or buproprion, even if the person does not meet the criteria for depression, as these agents are also sometimes helpful. Anecdotal reports have been published of the successful treatment of apathy with amantadine, bromocriptine, and selegiline. Apathy can be worsened by medications known to blunt emotion or slow cognitive processing, such as neuroleptics or benzodiazepines.

Nonpharmacologic Approaches to Treating Apathy

While apathetic individuals have trouble initiating actions, they will often participate if someone else sets up the activity and works along with them to sustain energy and attention. Maintaining a regular schedule, increasing environmental stimulation, such as involvement in a day program, avoiding open-ended questions or tasks, and providing cues may also help.

Case Study: #3

The Psychiatric Disorder: Apathy

A man with a five year history of HD no longer works and spends most of his waking time watching television. On his birthday, his brother arrived unexpectedly to take him fishing. Fishing had always been one of the man's favorite activities. The man initially declines to go until prodded by his brother and his wife. On the lake, the man seems more his usual self and catches several fish. On their return, however, he shows no interest in cleaning the fish, does not want to talk about his day, and simply turns the television on. The brother brings him to the doctor because he has heard that depression is very common in people with HD.

When asked about his mood, the man says "fine." He is not self-critical or hopeless. He describes his energy as normal. He is not having any suicidal thoughts or feelings of wanting to die. He still enjoys television and never misses his favorite programs. He eats and sleeps normally. When the doctor asks why he did not want to go fishing, he replies "I just didn't care."

The doctor explains to the family that the man is experiencing apathy, not depression. Both are common symptoms of HD. When pressed by the family to prescribe a treatment, the doctor explains that while there may be a few medications which could help, it is probably most important for the man's family and friends to understand his changing needs and to realize that apathy does not cause the man distress. The doctor suggests that a regular schedule of activities may be more helpful than spontaneous suggestions, and the man's family gets him enrolled in a three day a week morning activity program at the local veteran's center.

Perseveration and Fixation

People with HD tend to suffer from perseveration. This reduced mental and emotional flexibility may present as difficulty switching topics or letting go of an idea. Sometimes a person with HD will become fixated on a particular topic to the exclusion of almost all other concerns. Oftentimes this will be triggered by some loss of autonomy, and the preoccupation will revolve around something like the restoration of driving privileges, the ability to go hunting with shotguns, or control of finances. Other times the topic will be less predictable, an imagined slight, an unfulfilled responsibility, a financial concern, or animosity toward an acquaintance or neighbor. Distraction may help and sometimes the fixation diminishes over time.

Management of Perseveration or Fixation

When dealing with fixations, the family should be encouraged to "pick their battles." Confrontations should be saved for situations having to do with safety. This will be an easier point to get across if the family understands that these behaviors are due to the HD itself and that their loved one cannot "be reasonable."

Non-pharmacological management includes behavioral modification strategies and family education. Referral to a psychologist may be helpful. The physician can try treatment with SSRIs for their possible anti-obsessive effect. There is some theoretical basis for a dopamine-augmenting strategy in the treatment of executive dysfunction. There have been several cases of successful treatment with amantadine.

Case Study: #4

The Psychiatric Disorder: Perseveration

Mary is a 45 year old married woman with moderate HD. She and her husband arrive late for their appointment at the clinic. Her husband explains that lately she has become preoccupied with fruit juice. She demands that he keep six different kinds stocked in the refrigerator and will demand a glass of a specific juice to the exclusion of all other activities. On the morning of this visit, as they were supposed to leave for the two-hour trip to the clinic, she demanded that he go back into the house and bring her a glass of orange-pineapple juice. He refused and she had been haranguing him for the entire two hour journey and is still in a very bad mood. When asked how she is feeling today, she replies "I would be feeling better if my husband had given me the right kind of juice." "I will hear about this the entire trip home," her husband comments grimly.

Irritability

Irritability is a common complaint from people with HD and their families. Irritability can be a symptom of depression, but irritability occurring without a known cause reflects a loss of the ability of the brain to regulate the experience and expression of emotion. It may take the form of an increase in the person's baseline level of irritability, or there may be episodes of explosiveness as irritable responses to life events become exaggerated in intensity and duration. Some individuals, who are not irritable under most circumstances, will develop a kind of rigidity of thinking which will cause them to perseverate relentlessly on a particular desire or idea, becoming progressively angrier if their demands are not met (see perseveration).

People with HD may exhibit the "hypofrontal" condition of impaired control over behavior resulting from an imbalance between impulse and reflection. They may not be responsive to reason or inclined to back down from a conflict. Therefore, management of irritability consists primarily of identifying the situations that cause conflict. By working to avoid known triggers, caregivers can reduce head to head conflict and clinicians can avoid premature or excessive use of medications.

Irritability in the Home Environment

When irritability is severe, or enduring, or is expressed physically, caregivers may ask the physician to prescribe something to "calm him down." In such situations, the doctor needs to begin a careful review of the HD person's behavior, both as observed during the office visit and as reported by the family or caregivers. What does the informant really mean by saying the person is irritable or agitated? What behaviors has the person with HD exhibited? Symptoms could include restlessness, yelling or verbal abuse, explosive emotional outbursts, or physically violent behavior. How often has this behavior occurred and are there specific events that trigger it? It can be very helpful for the caregiver to create a log or diary of these events to support treatment decisions.

Understanding Irritability in HD

Many factors can precipitate an irritable episode, such as hunger, pain, inability to communicate, frustration with failing capabilities, boredom, and changes in expected routine. Some outbursts have no apparent cause and should be considered a consequence of the disease itself.

Due to the changes in brain function, confrontations and ultimatums are rarely productive. Family members and caregivers can be counseled to respond diplomatically and encouraged to understand that the HD person's irritability is a symptom of the disease. Irritability may be reduced if the environment is kept as calm and structured as possible. Family settings in which there are children and adolescents, unpredictable working hours, noise, or general chaos may worsen irritability and aggressiveness in people with HD. Caretaker and family support groups can provide emotional support and are a forum for sharing strategies that members have found useful in their own households.

Treating Irritability

For episodic outbursts, success often results from combining drug therapy with a careful analysis of the context and precipitants of the outburst. A number of medications have been found to be helpful in treating enduring irritability. People with HD may respond to antidepressants, particularly the SSRIs (sertraline, fluoxetine, and paroxetine), even if they do not meet all the criteria for major depression. The optimal doses for treating irritability are not known but one should start at a low dose and increase gradually as in the treatment of depression. These agents may be particularly useful when the irritability seems tied to the person's obsessive preoccupation with a particular topic. As in the treatment of depression, improvement may not occur for several weeks.

In severe or urgent situations most clinicians would probably start with a neuroleptic, particularly one of the newer agents which tend to have fewer side effects. Long-acting benzodiazepines, such as clonazepam (Klonopin®), starting at low doses, e.g. 0.5 mg/day, have also been helpful. The clinician must carefully monitor people with HD who are treated with these agents, as overdosing might lead to a mishap such as a fall or aspiration. Mood stabilizers, such as divalproex sodium and other anticonvulsants, have also been helpful and could be administered as outlined for mania.

Irritability, Outbursts and Safety

Family members and caregivers should be advised to avoid situations which could compromise safety. Walking away from an argument, leaving the room or even the premises to give the person with HD time to calm down may sometimes be necessary to avoid a physical altercation. The first priority is to ensure the immediate safety of the person and the caregiver. In cases of serious threat or actual violence, the caregiver should summon police, even if he or she does not intend to file charges, and should explain to the responders that the individual is suffering from a neuropsychiatric disease and is under a doctor's care. The responders will be able to control the immediate situation and assist the person with HD in receiving emergency evaluation and care. In some situations, the caregiver may actually want to consider allowing charges to be filed. This may help to reinforce the unacceptability of violence to a person who still retains some insight, or may permit a judge to compel treatment in someone who has previously been resisting it.

Psychiatric Problems not Belonging to a Distinct Category

Delirium

Delirium is an abnormal change in an HD person's level of consciousness, which may result from a variety of toxic, structural or metabolic causes. Delirious individuals may have waxing and waning of consciousness, may be agitated or lethargic, and frequently have disturbed sleep. It may also be accompanied by hallucinations or paranoia. People with HD are particularly vulnerable to delirium, especially in the later stages.

Common causes of delirium in HD include prescription medications, particularly benzodiazepines and anti-cholinergic agents, alcohol or illicit drugs, and medical problems such as dehydration and respiratory or urinary tract infections.

Delirium in HD may be misidentified as depression. Clinicians usually expect delirious individuals to exhibit agitation or hyper-arousal, and may overlook the delirious person who is somnolent or obtunded. Physicians should consider a diagnosis of delirium whenever confronted with an acute behavioral change in someone with HD and should review the medication list, examine the person, and obtain necessary laboratory studies, including a toxicology screen if indicated.

It is important to ask about over the counter medicines such as cold tablets and sleep aids, which individuals and families may forget to mention, and which may have negative interactions with other medications the person with HD is taking. Subdural hematoma, due to a recognized or unrecognized fall, should also be considered if the person suffers a sudden change in mental status. Delirium may come about gradually as the result of an undiagnosed underlying problem. For example, a dehydrated individual may no longer be able to tolerate his usual medication regimen.

Identification and correction of the underlying cause is the definitive treatment for delirium. Low doses of neuroleptics may be helpful in managing the agitation of a delirious individual temporarily.

Case Study: #5

The Psychiatric Disorder: Delirium

The husband of a 55 year old woman with moderate HD calls the HD clinic to ask about a change in her condition. "She seems confused today," he reports, "and she keeps falling asleep while I am trying to talk to her." He wants to know if this is an expected aspect of her Huntington's Disease. The doctor reminds him that "nothing changes suddenly in HD" and that the woman sounds delirious. The doctor explains that three very common causes of delirium in a person with HD are urinary tract infection, pneumonia, and subdural hematoma. The husband says that his wife falls a lot and could have hit her head in an unwitnessed accident. The doctor advises him to take his wife to an emergency room for tests. A very large subdural hematoma is discovered by CT scan, the hematoma is surgically evacuated, and the woman is sitting up and feeding herself a hearty breakfast by the next morning.

Anxiety

Anxiety is not a single syndrome, but serves as the final common pathway for many different psychiatric disorders. Some people with HD will experience anxiety because of challenging life circumstances, because of physical changes in the brain, and because of the interplay of the two. For example, some may develop social anxiety in response to their visible symptoms. Later in the course of the disease, as thought processes become less flexible, people with HD may be made anxious by trivial departures from their usual routine, such as an unexpected visitor or a delayed meal. They may worry for days in advance about what to wear when going to an appointment or what to order at a restaurant.

Treating Anxiety in HD

To address anxiety in a non-pharmacological manner, attempts should be made to decrease the complexity of the individual's environment. Choices and decisions should be simplified as much as possible. Stopping a job that has become too difficult may result in a remarkable improvement. Encouraging the caregiver to establish a predictable routine for the person with HD is often very helpful. Some caregivers find it useful to refrain from discussing any anxiety provoking events until the day before they are to occur. People with HD, who are very fearful of going to the doctor, may need to be told only that they are going on an errand until they reach the clinic.

Some individuals will not improve with counseling and environmental interventions and will require pharmacotherapy. The clinician should first assess whether the anxiety is a symptom of some other psychiatric condition, such as a major depression. People with obsessive compulsive disorder may be made anxious by obsessions or if their rituals are interrupted. Common agents for anxiety include the SSRI antidepressants, the benzodiazepines, and non-benzodiazepine anxiolytics such as buspirone.

Panic Disorder

Panic disorder is relatively uncommon in HD, but highly treatable. It is characterized by the acute onset of overwhelming anxiety and dread, accompanied by physiological symptoms such as rapid heartbeat, sweating, hyperventilation, light-headedness, or paraesthesias. Panic attacks usually last only fifteen or twenty minutes, may begin during sleep, and may even result in synocope (tingling or creeping feeling in the skin). Suspected panic attacks require medical evaluation, because some of the other possible explanations for the symptoms are dangerous conditions. Once these other causes have been ruled out, the usual treatment consists of SSRIs, sometimes temporarily supplemented with benzodiazepines. SSRIs are usually mildly stimulating and should be initiated at the lowest dose. Benzodiazepines should be used judiciously in the anxious person with HD because of the vulnerability of these people to delirium and falls, and because of their potential for abuse, especially in those whose judgment may already be impaired. These medications may have to be controlled by a family member. Some people with HD will respond to the non-benzodiazepine anxiolytic buspirone, which can be started at 5 mg two to three times per day and advanced to 20-30 mg per day in divided doses.

Sexual Problems

HD can cause a variety of changes in sexual behavior. The most common sexual problem is a loss of interest in sexual activity. This may occur fairly early in the course of the disease, when the individual is still functional in most other ways and can be very frustrating for the spouse or partner. Other people with HD may continue to enjoy sexual activity well into the course of the illness.

Issues of sexual incompatibility may also arise between the person with HD and their sexual partner. The partner may no longer think of the person in a sexual way, or they may find that the changes in appearance or mannerisms caused by HD make sex awkward or unappealing. Frank discussion with each person, individually and together, may help to improve understanding and generate compromises. Occasionally, in relation to personality changes and loss of inhibitions, a person with HD may desire and pursue excessive sexual activity or engage in new or inappropriate sexual behaviors, such as public masturbation, or voyeurism. The spouse, usually the wife, may be distressed and apprehensive that the person will become aggressive if sexual demands are not met. Spouses may be afraid to talk about the problem unless interviewed alone. Open communication about sex between the doctor and the family can help to de-stigmatize this sensitive topic, and distressing sexual behaviors can sometimes be adapted into more acceptable acts. Interventions can be difficult in circumstances where impaired judgment is an issue. Anti-androgenic therapy has been found to be helpful in a few of these cases.

Sleep Problems

Insomnia in people with HD may have a number of causes, including chorea, lack of daytime stimulation, depression, apathy or deterioration of the sleep-wake cycle. Generally speaking, chorea in HD tends to fade during sleep, but may make it difficult for the person to fall asleep in the first place, or to go back to sleep after a nighttime awakening. A formal sleep study can be useful for confirmation. In such cases, bedtime use of drugs to suppress chorea may solve the problem.

Keeping the individual awake and active, for example through a day program, may be all that is needed to counteract under-stimulation and achieve restful sleep.

Depressed individuals commonly complain of early morning awakening or may appear to sleep most of the night but not feel rested in the morning. Those complaining of insomnia should be asked about other symptoms of depression.

There are no ideal hypnotic medications, but agents such as sedating antidepressants (such as trazodone) or neuroleptics (such as quetiapine) may be used judiciously. Benzodiazepine and other prescription sedative-hypnotics are potentially delirogenic and habit forming and should be used cautiously, if at all.

Apathetic people with HD often sleep excessively or spend an inordinate amount of time in bed. This may be acceptable to the person and family if it is understood as a feature of the disease. Enrollment in a regular activity program, organized by others, can be an effective intervention for the apathetic person with HD. In situations where harm could result from apathy, for example if the person is not getting out of bed for meals, judicious use of amphetamines may be appropriate.

Demoralization

People with HD may become demoralized at various times during their illness, particularly when meaningful losses accumulate over a short period of time, such as the loss of a job, control of one's finances or driving privileges. The person experiences the failure of his hopes for the future and the loss of his sense of self worth and begins to experience despair. People with HD may remain fixated on their losses resulting in hospitalizations and suicide attempts. Demoralization should be considered when the person lacks the full depressive syndrome, and when the feelings of hopelessness have arisen in clear proximity to significant losses.

Treatment for demoralization requires a combination of psychotherapy and social work to help the individual, and his or her family, solve real world problems, reduce stressors, build a support system, and emphasize the positive factors in life.

Psychiatric Disorder: Demoralization

A 48 year-old married man with very mild Huntington's Disease has been forced to divulge his diagnosis and take disability from his job as a police officer when he is no longer able to qualify on the gun range. His disability pension is fairly generous and his wife picks up extra hours at her job to make ends meet. Now that he is home, however, he is not helping with the household chores, is irritable with his wife and children and is beginning to drink excessively in the evenings. He tells his wife that he feels worthless and "half a man" and she is worried because he still owns a revolver.

The doctor asks him directly if he has been having suicidal thoughts. He seems surprised at the question and replies that he would never do such a thing to hurt his family. He discusses his feelings of guilt and worthlessness over not being able to provide for his family.

The doctor reminds him that his condition is very mild and that he has many good years ahead of him. He agrees to abstain from alcohol for the time being and, with encouragement, obtains a part time job providing security at a large retail store. He is open about his condition and is not required to carry a gun. With the money he is making, his wife is able to reduce her hours and now that he is feeling less resentful, he begins to pitch in at home, going grocery shopping or doing the laundry.

He starts to meet weekly with a social worker at the HD clinic and he and his wife begin to attend a monthly HD support group. Six months later, at a follow-up visit, he is in excellent spirits and has made a successful transition to his new situation.

Chapter 7

Juvenile Onset
Huntington's Disease

Martha Nance, M.D.

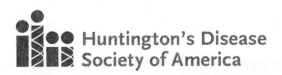
**Huntington's Disease
Society of America**

Juvenile Onset Huntington's Disease

Fewer than ten percent of people with Huntington's Disease (HD) develop symptoms before age 20[1]. Juvenile onset HD (JHD) presents unique challenges to affected individuals, their caregivers, and the various professionals who are called upon to assist them.

Diagnosing JHD is not an easy task. Symptoms of JHD are often the same as symptoms of other conditions, and while there is a genetic test for the mutated HD gene, genetic testing must be used with particular caution in children, as the presence of the HD gene in a blood test does not necessarily mean that the child's symptoms are due to Huntington's Disease. HDSA strongly recommends that the family or physician contact an HDSA Center of Excellence or a genetic counselor familiar with HD to discuss a specific child or situation in more detail before a genetic test is performed.

When to Consider Juvenile onset HD

The presenting symptoms of Huntington's Disease may be a little different in a child than in an adult, particularly a child under 10 years of age. While there is no symptom or group of symptoms that are absolutely required for the diagnosis of JHD, most affected children have several of the features described (see box) at the time that the diagnosis is made.

Chorea is uncommon in children developing HD within the first decade, but may be one of the first symptoms in a teenager. Severe behavioral disturbances may be the first symptom in an adolescent.

Typical Initial Symptoms of Juvenile onset HD

- Positive family history of HD, usually in the father

- Stiffness of the legs

- Clumsiness of arms and legs

- Decline in cognitive function

- Changes in behavior

- Seizures

- Changes in oral motor function

- Chorea in an adolescent

- Behavioral disturbances

---

1   Harper, P.S. 1996 *Huntington's Disease,* 2nd Edition. WB Saunders: London

Family History

For reasons that only became clear after the gene responsible for HD was discovered in 1993, children with a very early onset of HD are more likely to have an affected father than an affected mother. It is very unlikely for HD to appear in a child whose parent was not also affected with HD. If this situation appears to be present, the physician should consider diagnoses other than HD. Occasionally, there may be an HD-affected child without an apparently affected parent. This may be due to the onset of symptoms in the child before the parent's onset, the early death of a parent (before the parent's symptoms were evident), misdiagnosis or lack of diagnosis in a parent who was affected, non-paternity (a biological father who is not the same as the apparent father), or adoption. Documenting the diagnosis of HD in other relatives can be helpful to the physician as the child is evaluated for HD.

Movement Disorders

The most visible symptoms of HD are related to movement. HD can cause involuntary movements, or chorea, and also affect control over voluntary movement. Children who show HD symptoms before the age of 10, however, often present with rigidity and may never experience chorea, whereas those who develop the disease as adolescents may display chorea as an early symptom.

Rigidity

A child with JHD will likely exhibit difficulties with balance and walking, as well as clumsiness of hand and arm movements, thickness of speech, drooling, and poor oral motor control. Toe-walking and scissoring of gait are particularly common in younger children.

Chorea

Chorea, which is a term for the involuntary jerking or twitching movements which often appear in adult onset HD, is rarely found in Juvenile onset HD that appears before age 10, but may cause difficulties for adolescents with the disease. Choreiform movements may be small or large in amplitude, manifesting as finger flicking, shoulder shrugging, facial grimacing and flailing of the arms or legs. Chorea may also contribute to difficulty with speaking, chewing, and swallowing. Chorea can interfere with the saccadic movements of the eyes needed for reading.

Declining Cognitive Function

Because HD is a degenerative condition, affected children will begin to lose skills that they had previously gained. In a school-aged child, this is often noticed first as an overall decline in grades or other measures of school performance. Attention and concentration may decline, frequently leading to a diagnosis of attention deficit disorder (ADD). Of course, ADD is a common condition that can certainly be present in a child who does not have HD.

In a younger child, increasing difficulty with previously attained cognitive or motor skills, such as speech, reading, math, throwing a ball, swimming or riding a bicycle, might be evident. In a young child or pre-teenager, the combination of declining school performance, along with worsening motor skills, would be more suggestive of HD than a change in grades alone.

In an adolescent, many other common causes of poor school performance must be considered, including depression, attention deficit disorder, learning disabilities, drug or alcohol use, or disruptions of family or social life. Detailed information from teachers and school counselors may help the physician to pinpoint the different kinds and causes of dysfunction at school.

Behavioral Disturbance

Behavioral disturbances are common in children with HD. However, behavioral disturbances, depression, and attention deficit disorder/hyperactivity are also common in children without HD. The family of a child at-risk for HD is often under significant financial and social stress because a parent or sibling is already affected by the disease. This family stress increases the chance of social and behavioral problems in the child.

In younger children, when aggressive or disruptive behavior is related to HD, it is usually seen along with changes in cognitive function and motor disturbance. In adolescents, behavioral disturbance may be the first and only presenting symptom of HD. Behavior problems in adolescents with HD are often very severe, leading to psychiatric hospitalization, suspension from school, or involvement with law enforcement agencies. Examples have included arson, theft, sexual promiscuity, physical or sexual abuse of younger siblings, severe drug or alcohol abuse, and depression with suicide attempts.

Seizures

Seizures are said to occur in about 25% of children with Juvenile onset HD, and may be a presenting symptom. They may be of any type, and they may or may not be severe. The physician can never simply assume that the seizures are caused by HD; any child with a seizure should have cerebral imaging studies and an electro-encephalogram (EEG), as well as appropriate laboratory studies, to rule out metabolic causes such as low blood sugar or drug or toxin ingestion.

Initial Consultation

The diagnosis of Juvenile onset HD can be challenging, especially to a physician unfamiliar with the condition, and a diagnosis is unlikely to be made during the first visit. The family should be apprised of the steps involved in making the diagnosis and prepared for the amount of time it may take to determine whether the symptoms the child is experiencing are caused by JHD or some other disease or combination of disorders.

Children in HD families can have developmental delay, attention deficit disorder, mental retardation, or other medical or neurological conditions entirely unrelated to HD. Brain imaging, by computerized tomography (CT) or magnetic resonance imaging (MRI), is often normal early in the course of HD but may be helpful to rule out other conditions. Similarly, routine blood tests, while not helpful in securing a diagnosis of HD, can help to rule out other diseases that can cause abnormal movements, such as hyper- or hypothyroidism, toxin or drug ingestion, systemic lupus erythematosus, or recent streptococcal infection (Sydenham's chorea).

A referral to a pediatric neurologist or HD specialist may be part of obtaining a diagnosis. Because JHD is a rare condition, an adult neurologist specializing in movement disorders or HD may be more helpful than a pediatric neurologist who is unfamiliar with the condition. The regional HDSA Center of Excellence can help you locate a neurologist in the area who is familiar with the condition.

If cognitive changes are present, a formal neuropsychological assessment (tests of memory, developmental skills, and intelligence) can document areas of strength and weakness, suggest strategies for management and serve as a baseline for comparison later. The neuropsychologist should also review, along with the physician, any previous records of neurological exams, psychological evaluations, or school testing, looking for the declines that would suggest that a degenerative process is ongoing. Physical, occupational, and speech-language pathologists can perform baseline assessments of motor skills with an emphasis on how the child is able to function in school and at home.

Based on the at-risk child's behavior and school performance, the physician may also need to evaluate the child's psychosocial situation to make appropriate referrals for individual or family counseling, county-based child protective services, school-based programs, or social services.

Genetic Testing for Juvenile onset HD

When the history, examination, and initial laboratory evaluation are strongly suggestive of HD, a genetic test may be the most efficient and accurate way to confirm the diagnostic impression. On the other hand, the decision to perform a genetic test on a child is a complex and emotional one for families. A positive test result in the setting of symptoms unrelated to HD (headaches and blurry vision, for instance, or isolated attention deficit disorder), may result in the failure to identify an unrelated medical condition (such as a pituitary tumor), and the erroneous assignment of the symptoms to HD, while constituting a predictive gene test done without the child's understanding or consent.

It is recommended that the neurologist evaluate the child twice, six to twelve months apart. If the initial symptoms have remained or progressed despite optimal management, then it may be appropriate to do the HD gene test at the time of the second visit. This strategy makes it less likely that a child with temporary or non-progressive symptoms would be tested prematurely, while avoiding the multi-year delay in diagnosis that families often observe.

The diagnosis of Juvenile onset HD, whether based on a clinical examination alone, or secured with a gene test, will give an explanation for symptoms that may have confused and frightened the child and the family. This may relieve stress and minimize "acting out" on the part of the child.

A firm diagnosis also gives the family and doctors a more clear direction regarding the prognosis and care. Thus, it is equally important for the physician to make a diagnosis of Juvenile onset HD in a timely fashion, and not to postpone or refuse genetic confirmation of the diagnosis in a child whose symptoms and course suggest that the diagnosis of Juvenile onset HD is quite likely.

After the Diagnosis

The Expected Course

Juvenile onset HD is a chronic, terminal condition that typically progresses over a number of years. Some children, particularly those with a very young age of onset, follow a more rapid disease course over a shorter number of years. There is no way to predict, at the onset of the disease, which child is likely to have a longer or shorter disease duration.

In late stage JHD, the affected child (who by then may be an adult) will require 24-hour supervision and extensive assistance with the daily activities of life. Swallowing and communication problems are universal in late stage HD. Death in JHD, unless it occurs unexpectedly due to accident or injury, is preceded by a time when the young person is increasingly unable to communicate or eat safely.

At the present time, there is no cure and no medication that is known to slow down the progression of the disease. The goals of treatment in JHD, as in adult onset HD, are to reduce the burden of symptoms, maximize function and optimize quality of life.

Team Based Care

Treating a child with HD requires a creative, global approach by a team of doctors and allied healthcare professionals: a neurologist, psychologist or psychiatrist, a physical therapist, occupational therapist and speech-language pathologist, as well as the primary care physician and dentist who take care of the child's general medical and dental health. The recommendations presented in Chapter 3, Team Based Care, are applicable to the care of a child with HD.

The role of the lead physician will be to coordinate care and to manage the symptoms that can be treated in order to promote optimal functioning and quality of life for the child. The physician can help the family set reasonable goals and expectations and plan ahead for the changes that occur during the course of the disease, so that they do not come as a surprise.

Understanding the Interrelated Disorders of HD

The core features of HD in a child or an adult are 1) the movement disorder (difficulty with movement), 2) the cognitive disorder (dementia), and 3) behavior and psychiatric issues (mood or behavior changes). Problems or declining abilities in one area will affect other areas. Each symptom must be looked at and treated within the context of interrelated disabilities.

Progression of the *Movement Disorder*

Children who show symptoms of HD before age 10 often develop rigidity or spasticity of the trunk or limbs. Initially, this is often most severe in the legs. The child may begin to walk on his/her toes, lose control of balance when running, hopping, or bicycling, or develop a scissoring or stiff-legged gait. Older children (teenagers) with HD may develop chorea – the involuntary, irregular, fidgety or jerky movements of the arms, legs, trunk, neck, or face that are one of the most common symptoms in adults.

Over time, children with HD have increasing difficulty controlling voluntary movements. There will be a progressive loss of oral motor function, which can cause slurring of speech, difficulty swallowing, or drooling. Clumsiness becomes noticeable, and the child may have difficulty with previously learned skills, such as throwing a ball or writing. As the disease progresses, even simple single movements such as those needed to bathe or dress can be difficult, and awkward stiff postures of the limbs or trunk, called dystonia, may become severe.

Treatments and Therapies for the Movement Disorder

Physical therapy, occupational therapy and speech-language pathology may be very therapeutic throughout the course of the disease. A home assessment by a public health nurse or occupational therapist may be useful. He or she can perform a room-by-room assessment of safety and functionality, and make recommendations to the family for medical equipment or modifications which will improve the child's quality of life.

Early introduction of routines and devices is important with all therapies for children with JHD, beginning before it appears that the intervention or device is actually necessary. This is because cognitive decline is a major part of the disease. A child will be better able to learn how to use a new device or therapy if it is introduced while he/she is able to understand and cooperate. By the time the need for the device becomes more obvious, it is a familiar thing that can easily be incorporated into daily use.

Physical Therapy

The physical therapist can help throughout the course of the disease, addressing problems with body movements, such as walking, and movement in and out of a chair, bed, or car, as well as problems with posture, and muscle tone. Initially, all children diagnosed with Juvenile onset HD should have an age-appropriate activity program that emphasizes full range of motion of the limbs, trunk, and neck, and aerobic exercise. The physical therapist can help to develop this program.

Physical therapy consultation is particularly important for children with rigidity, spasticity, or dystonia. Splinting or bracing of a limb may improve function. Heat, stretching, and massage may help to relieve discomfort caused by dystonia.

Occupational Therapy

The occupational therapist often focuses on small movements and the performance of daily activities of life such as bathing, dressing, and eating, with an emphasis on safety and improved and independent function. In the early stages of the disease, an assessment can provide a baseline for later comparison, and can also alert the family to things that should be watched.

The therapist can also recommend adaptive equipment such as helmets and protective pads, walkers with wheels, and wheelchairs. As the disease progresses, special seating devices, cushions, mattresses, and padding may be needed to protect stiff limbs or joints and to prevent bruises or abrasions.

Speech-Language Pathology and Nutritional Consultation

The progressive loss of muscle control in JHD affects the ability to swallow and consume enough calories. A speech-language pathologist (SLP) and a nutritionist may be needed to address these difficulties. A speech-language pathologist can help the child with exercises to strengthen the chewing muscles and teach strategies for reducing the threat of choking while eating. A nutritionist can give the caregiver guidance on providing high-calorie foods that are easy to chew and swallow.

Medication for the Movement Disorder in JHD

No medications improve control of voluntary movements, although there are treatments for rigidity, spasticity, dystonia, and chorea that may help children with JHD. Medications for treating chorea are discussed in Chapter 4, The Motor Disorder, and in *The Juvenile HD Handbook: A Guide for Physicians, Neurologists and Other Professionals,* available on the HDSA website at www.hdsa.org.

The *Cognitive Disorder*

Like adults, young people with JHD may experience changes in memory, judgment and problem solving. Sometimes these problems start before physical symptoms of the disease appear.

JHD makes it difficult to organize incoming stimulus. A noisy room or complicated instructions can overwhelm the child and trigger outbursts of emotion or aggression. The child may have difficulty starting or completing a task, or trouble doing all the steps of a task in the right order. Symptoms may be misdiagnosed as inattention or hyperactivity, or be mistaken for "bad behavior," when in actuality it is the disease that is interfering with the child's ability to concentrate.

Medication for the Cognitive Disorder

No medications have been proven to improve cognitive function in HD. However, if frequent seizures, attention deficit, or depression are interfering with a child's ability to perform, treating these symptoms may improve the child's quality of life. Several medications are FDA-approved and widely used for the treatment of dementia in people with Alzheimer's disease (donepezil, rivastigmine, galantamine, and memantine), but none have been evaluated in more than a handful of adults with HD, and none can be recommended to treat Juvenile onset HD.

The *Behavioral and Psychiatric Disorders*

While the movement disorder can cause the most visible symptoms, changes in behavior may actually be among the earliest symptoms of Juvenile onset HD. Changes to the brain may alter the behavior of the child and can cause them to do things that seem completely "out of character." Many times, these emotional/ behavioral symptoms become a significant disability. In the case of adolescents, the behavioral disorders may become severe and dangerous.

Behavioral/Psychiatric Disorders common to both HD and JHD include:

- Depression, anxiety and guilt

- Irritability/agitation

- Emotional and temper outbursts

- Impulsive behavior/aggression

- Obsessive/paranoid thoughts

- Apathy/denial

- Rigid thinking

- Disorganization and/or forgetfulness

Depression

Depression is the most common mood disturbance in children with JHD. Particularly in a young child, who may not know the words to describe his/her feelings, depression may appear as a significant change in sleep habits (too much or too little), change in appetite or weight (in either direction), lack of interest in previously enjoyed activities, or poor performance at school. The behavioral disorders of JHD and the symptoms of depression can be confusingly similar.

A child with JHD experiencing a mild depression may respond to medication, while at other times counseling may be helpful, or the two can be used together. Severe depression requires a psychiatric specialist, and on rare occasions, even a young child may need hospitalization because he or she represents a threat to himself or others.

There are many medications that are effective in treating depression in people with HD. These medications and their potential side effects are discussed in Chapter 6, The Psychiatric Disorder. Further information on depression in JHD can be found in *The Juvenile HD Handbook: A Guide for Physicians, Neurologists and Other Professionals.*

Severely depressed individuals should be asked whether they have suicidal thoughts or plans. Asking about suicide does not plant the idea in the child's mind, but may provide a welcomed opportunity for the young person to discuss troubling thoughts.

Obsession

Obsessive thinking is a common symptom of Juvenile onset HD. When the thoughts of the affected child and the requests or plans of the caregiver come into conflict, aggressive behavior often results.

Behavioral modification strategies can be used to limit the disruptive behavior that can accompany obsession, or to restrict the activity to appropriate times or locations. Creating a limited outlet for the idea or obsession may be helpful for managing the symptom. A psychologist or psychiatrist is best equipped to help the family manage obsessive behavior.

Medication may be effective in suppressing obsessive thoughts. Further information can be found in *The Juvenile HD Handbook: A Guide for Physicians, Neurologists and Other Professionals.*

Behavior Management - Outbursts, Impulsiveness, Explosive or Violent Behavior

Behavior management represents the greatest challenge for JHD families. Mood swings and impulsiveness are common in children with JHD. In adolescents, these symptoms can escalate into dangerous behavior.

Damage to the basal ganglia will reduce impulse control in children with JHD and may lead to outbursts, aggressiveness or even violence. Children and youth in the middle or late stages of JHD often lack a sense of time. Memory can be so poor that the child doesn't recall that he had a soda or piece of candy fifteen minutes earlier. Parents may be advised to "pick their battles" and compromise if a situation begins to escalate toward a crisis. From the start, families should be encouraged to try to identify factors or situations that tend to trigger aggressive behaviors.

Some families may not be able to identify specific situations that trigger violent or aggressive behavior, or may not be able to control the behaviors using the techniques described above. In these instances, aggressive, impulsive, or violent children may need medications to help them control their behavior.

Mood stabilizing medications and their potential side effects are discussed in Chapter 6, The Psychiatric Disorder and in *The Juvenile HD Handbook: A Guide for Physicians, Neurologists and Other Professionals.*

Some children may have attention deficit disorder or hyperactivity in addition to JHD. For these children, treating these symptoms may lead to an improvement in behavior. Similarly, treating an underlying depression can lead to marked improvement in angry, aggressive, or dangerous behavior. However, medications alone cannot control behavior. The physician may recommend visits to a family counselor, child psychologist, or psychiatrist to help both the family and the child to understand and manage behavior problems better.

If a home situation is dangerous to the child or others in the family, a psychiatric hospitalization may be necessary. Removing the child temporarily allows both the child and the family to rest, reflect, and heal. The child can begin treatment in a safe environment, and the family can learn different ways to manage the situation when the child returns home.

Management of Other Disorders

Seizures

Seizures occur in about 25% of children with Juvenile onset HD, but are uncommon in those with adult-onset HD. This is probably because the developing brain of a child is more likely to develop seizures in response to an insult or injury than the adult brain.

The physician should never simply assume that seizures are caused by HD. Blood tests should be done to rule out an infection or problem with blood sugar, sodium, or other blood chemicals. In adolescents, screening the urine for toxins such as cocaine may be appropriate. All children with a first seizure should have a brain imaging test (preferably magnetic resonance imaging [MRI] rather than computerized tomography [CT] as it shows more detail), and an electro-encephalogram (EEG). The electrical characteristics of the seizures sometimes help to guide treatment.

Epilepsy often decreases in severity as the child grows older, so seizures that were once difficult to manage might become less of a problem later. There is not a particular time or stage of Juvenile onset HD when seizures are more likely to begin.

More information on seizures in Juvenile onset HD and treatment options is available in *The Juvenile HD Handbook: A Guide for Physicians, Neurologists and Other Professionals.*

Hallucinations

Hallucinations are uncommon in Juvenile onset HD, but do occur in occasional individuals. They can be auditory (such as hearing voices, which may simply make comments or may command the person to do something), visual, or sensory. They can occur in a person with severe depression, as a result of certain prescription medications, or because of the use of mind-altering drugs (such as stimulants or hallucinogens).

Medications to treat hallucinations are discussed in Chapter 6, The Psychiatric Disorder and in *The Juvenile HD Handbook: A Guide for Physicians, Neurologists and Other Professionals.*

Sexuality in Adolescents with JHD

Adolescence is a difficult time even for children who do not have HD. Managing a changing physical appearance, new and unfamiliar sexual urges, learning how to interact with peers who are undergoing similar changes, and moving away from relationships with parents into strong relationships with other adolescents and adults are tall tasks for any teenager. Facing these challenges, with a disease that diminishes the ability to communicate and to understand new information, and reduces the ability to suppress impulsive or disruptive behavior, is far more challenging.

Girls

For girls, a major challenge may be managing menstrual hygiene. Depending on how advanced JHD is when menses begin, gentle and repeated counseling and assistance from a trusted female relative or nurse may help the girl to understand the feelings that accompany menstruation, treatments that are available for bloating and menstrual cramps, and when and how to use menstrual hygiene products.

The physician should have a private discussion with the girl about what sexual activity includes, how to prevent pregnancy, when sexual activity is inappropriate, and how to obtain help if problems arise. Group discussions in a school health class may proceed too quickly for a girl with JHD to process all of the important information or to ask questions.

If appropriate, the physician should recommend contraceptive devices or medications for the girl with JHD. Contraceptive patches or long-acting injections may be preferable to pills or devices that must be used daily or at the time of a sexual encounter.

Depending on the social or clinical situation, some might consider a sterilization procedure. Early attention to these issues is important, as female adolescents with JHD may become sexually promiscuous without a real understanding of the potential consequences of their sexual activity. A public school may be obligated to provide a personal care attendant if a girl is judged to be particularly vulnerable to the sexual or physical advances of others.

Boys

Boys with JHD are also potentially vulnerable to sexual and physical abuse and to the consequences of their own impulsive or aggressive behavior. Boys who are teased or physically abused or threatened should be offered the same protection that vulnerable girls would be offered.

Boys who behave inappropriately may need both behavioral modification strategies and medications to manage their sexual urges and impulsive behaviors. For example, a boy who masturbates in public can be encouraged to use private areas such as the bedroom or bathroom, with the door closed, but may need medication if the inappropriate behavior continues or interferes with other daily activities.

Impulsive or aggressive sexual behaviors can be severe in adolescent boys with HD. Consultation with a psychiatrist or psychologist experienced in the management of sexual or conduct disorders may be helpful, and inpatient treatment may be appropriate in severe cases. Medication options for boys exhibiting aggressive sexual behavior can be found in *The Juvenile HD Handbook: A Guide for Physicians, Neurologists and Other Professionals*, available on the HDSA website, www.hdsa.org.

Staying Safe – Mental Illness and Juvenile onset HD

Juvenile onset HD can cause serious mental health conditions and even psychosis. As the disease progresses, the young person may become confused or act aggressively, even toward family members and siblings. Verbal abuse, threats, temper tantrums and even physical violence are a possibility.

Juvenile onset HD can cause a young person to become involved in dangerous behavior, or become unwilling to take needed medications. Early intervention and sustained treatment when symptoms of mental illness are present is essential to maintaining quality of life for the individual with Juvenile onset HD, their caregivers and the rest of the family.

Families should be encouraged to create a home management strategy to protect themselves in case of escalating aggressive or violent behavior by the child with JHD. They should be prepared with a safe room where they can go in time of crisis and to have a friend or neighbor who can be called upon to remove one or another party from the scene of the crisis. They should also be prepared to call for help from emergency services.

Caregivers of adolescents should consider creating an HD CARE Kit (Critical Advocacy Resources for Emergencies) which is a collection of documents and information that may be needed during a behavioral or psychiatric crisis. Explanation of and forms for a CARE kit may be found in Appendix VI of *The Juvenile HD Handbook: A Guide for Physicians, Neurologists and Other Professionals.*

A Functional Scale for the Stages of Juvenile onset HD

The following is a modification of the Shoulson-Fahn Functional Capacity Scale. Although this scale has not been scientifically validated, it may be clinically useful in judging how a child's HD is progressing. More information on this scale may be found in *The Juvenile HD Handbook: A Guide for Physicians, Neurologists and Other Professionals.*

While the scale may be useful in guiding treatment plans and informing the Individualized Education Plan (IEP) in the school, it does not account well for severe behavioral or psychiatric problems. Children and youth with early HD who have very severe behavior problems may score more poorly than their mental or motor skills would suggest, and improvement in the apparent disease stage could be seen if the severe behavior problems respond to treatment.

Stages of JHD (total points in all areas)

11-13 points	Stage 1
7-10 points	Stage 2
3-6 points	Stage 3
1-2 points	Stage 4
0 points	Stage 5

A. School attendance
3 – attends school, no special assistance needed
2 – attends school, some regular classes, some special or modified classes
1 – attends school, few or no regular classes
0 – unable to attend school or work program

B. Academic/developmental performance
3 – reading/writing/math skills appropriate to age
2 – mild decrease in academic performance but still able to take a test or to write
1 – unable to write legibly but able to communicate orally
0 – unable to read/write/communicate orally

C. Chores
2 – able to assist in age-appropriate manner with household chores
1 – occasionally assists with chores
0 – unable to participate in household chores

D. Activities of daily living
3 – performs self-cares in an age-appropriate manner
2 – requires some assistance for bathing, dressing, grooming, or feeding
1 – assists others who bathe, dress, or feed him/her
0 – unable to assist in self-cares

E. Lives
2 – at home with only family assistance
1 – at home/group home/foster care with assistance from non-family members
0 – living in a long-term care facility

The child with JHD will need a wide range of assistance to thrive in school and the family physician can play a vital role in helping the child to receive the assistance they are guaranteed under the Americans with Disabilities Act (ADA). An educational CD-ROM, *JHD in the School Environment*, is available from the HDSA National Office, 800 345-HDSA.

Caring for the Family Facing JHD

A family in which there is a child with Juvenile onset HD is a family under stress. Professional counseling should be made available to all family members before the situation becomes unmanageable. Many families facing JHD find it helpful if the entire family has regular visits with a family counselor.

Other Children

JHD affects the entire family. While it is not necessary to describe the late stages of the disease to a child whose brother or sister has just been diagnosed, it is important to address basic misunderstandings and fears that young children may have about JHD. As they grow up, siblings of a child with HD will gain an increasing awareness of their own risk of developing HD. It is important to make sure siblings have an accurate understanding of their risk of developing HD, but it is not necessary to over-emphasize it.

All children in an HD family, whether they have the disease or not, are at-risk for depression or stress-related problems. Counseling and support groups may be helpful. Many HDSA chapters offer support groups in locations across the U.S. These support groups can be found on the HDSA website, www.hdsa.org.

When a child moves into adolescence and has the potential to be sexually active, it is good to review how the HD gene is passed on from parent to child. Once an at-risk child has become an adult, and is able to make his/her own medical decisions, he or she can consider undergoing a gene test to determine whether the HD gene is present or not.

Late Stage HD and End of Life Issues

Although it is difficult to discuss the progression of symptoms or the late stages of a child's disease, it is important to do so. By having a realistic idea of the challenges ahead, parents or other caregivers have the time to ask questions, make plans, clear up any misunderstandings, and avoid surprises or crisis situations.

Issues that need to be discussed include the use of feeding tubes, hydration (fluids), antibiotics, hospitalization and resuscitation. The need for professional nursing, out of home placement, Advance Directives, medical Powers of Attorney and Hospice care are other important topics that may require family action.

A chaplain, minister, counselor, social worker, or nurse can help the physician to discuss end of life issues with the family. The goal is to help parents or caregivers to consider the issues and make decisions before a crisis emerges.

There is extensive information on late stage JHD and end of life issues in *The Juvenile HD Handbook: A Guide for Physicians, Neurologists and Other Professionals.*

Case Study: #1

Juvenile onset HD: Diagnosis

A 40 year old woman brings her 12 year old son to the clinic. The child's father, her ex-husband, has HD, but no longer lives in the home. This son, the oldest of 4 siblings, has been irritable and angry, with declining school performance over the last year. She thinks he has been using illicit drugs, because he is clumsy. She wants him to be tested for HD, because she is sure that he is symptomatic.

The examination shows some subtle motor abnormalities ("soft signs"), but the examining neurologist, not having examined the child before, feels that they could be in the range of normal for the child's age and developmental stage, and that the motor diagnosis of HD is not yet clear. Rather than order a confirmatory gene test, since the diagnosis is not yet clear, he orders formal cognitive testing and a baseline MRI scan. A pediatric psychiatrist is consulted, as well as a family counselor. The possibility (but lack of certainty) that these symptoms represent early HD is discussed with the mother, along with an emphasis on the management of the symptoms, whether or not the child will prove to have HD. Appropriate personnel from the school are involved in creating an educational plan based on the psychiatric diagnosis.

When the boy returns for follow up 6 months later, dystonia, eye movement abnormalities and clumsiness have become more evident, and the clinical diagnosis of HD is made. A confirmatory gene test shows one allele with 18 CAG repeats and the second with 61 CAG repeats, consistent with the clinical diagnosis of HD.

The family is informed about the diagnosis and the expected course and treatments. The boy will continue to receive care for his behavioral issues from the psychiatrist. The mother has already joined an on-line community of parents caring for children with JHD.

Chapter 8

Management of Late Stage HD

Martha Nance, M.D.

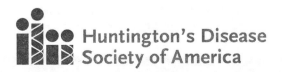
Huntington's Disease
Society of America

Management of Late Stage HD

The late stages of Huntington's Disease (HD) occupy a number of years, even a decade or more, of the life of a person with the disease. There are no evidence-based algorithms to guide the physician in providing sensitive and patient-oriented care in this difficult stage of the disease, but there are some common sense approaches which are outlined in this chapter. Until a cure is found for HD, it is incumbent upon the healthcare team to do all that it can to optimize function and quality of life for people with HD, from the beginning of the disease until the end.

In comparison to Alzheimer's disease, which progresses in a relatively uniform fashion over a short number of years, Huntington's Disease typically progresses over 10-20 years after diagnosis, and can follow one of several trajectories. Some people with HD have terribly chaotic lives, marked by severe behavioral disarray, requiring heavy involvement of local psychiatric, social, protective, legal, and judicial services, and exhausting or estranging themselves from family and friends. Others may have little or no mood disturbance, but severe chorea and gait disturbance. Still others may have significant unawareness or denial of symptoms, leading to inappropriate decisions or behaviors.

These general disease patterns, and others, persist into the late stages of the disease, so that there is not a single "snapshot" of late stage HD that fits all individuals. In addition, the degree to which people with HD have exhausted their personal or family resources (financial, logistical, and emotional), as well as community resources (day programs, in-home nursing services, long-term care facilities) can vary from person to person. Below is a general framework that should help health professionals to provide sensitive and personalized care to people who are reaching the most debilitating phase of their disease.

Defining "late stage" Huntington's Disease

Late stage HD can be characterized by the need for 24-hour supervision and care. People at this stage of HD are dependent on others for feeding, toileting and mobility. They may become unable to speak words, but still be able to communicate. Late stage HD is the time when out of home placement typically occurs. People with HD can live for 5 years or more after placement in a long-term care facility. Individuals, families, treating physicians, and staff at long-term care facilities need to plan for several years of disease management during the late stages of the disease.

People with HD who are judged to be in Stage 4 or 5 (0-2 points), according to the Shoulson-Fahn Total Functional Capacity Scale (TFC), are in the late stage of their disease. As people with HD are said to decline by 0.7 points on this 13-point scale each year, an average person with HD might reach the late stages about 10-15 years after diagnosis (depending on what the functional score was at the time of diagnosis).

Assessing Disease Progression during the Late Stages

Table 1 outlines a system for evaluating functional capacity in late stage HD, modeled after the TFC. This "Advanced HD Functional Capacity Scale" evaluates people along several domains: mobility, feeding, continence, communication, and interaction/participation. Although the scale has not been validated clinically, it might be useful to the care team as a guide to the kinds of functional changes that take place as a person progresses through the late stages of HD.

Table 1.

	Mobility	Feeding	Continence	Communication	Participation
	Advanced HD Functional Capacity Scale				
4	Walks, may have missteps, but no more than occasional falls			Communicates with people other than family, caregivers	Able to participate actively in family/ residence activities
3	Frequent falls or very frequent near falls	Eats independently, using at least a fork or spoon	Continent of both stool and urine, takes care of toilet hygiene	Phrases or sentences only intelligible to family or in context	Able to participate in some or occasional activities
2	Wheelchair, independent	Uses a cup/straw, finger foods	Not always continent, or poor toilet hygiene	Single words or severe dysarthria; limited ability to speak even with family or in context	Able to attend some activities but little or no active participation
1	Able to sit but dependent on others for mobility	Must be fed	Incontinent most or all of the time but aware	Mute but attempts to communicate (grunts, screams)	Able to respond interactively in some way to others
0	Bed-bound or unable to sit	Most or all nutrition provided by feeding tube	Incontinent and unaware or passive about help	Mute	Non-interactive

Maximum score 18 points, minimum score 0 points

Stage A1: 16-18 points (largely independent)

Stage A2: 10-15 points (still trying to be independent but not very successful)

Stage A3: 6-9 points (receives assistance with all activities but at least interacts)

Stage A4: 2-5 points (requires full assistance with everything)

Stage A5: 0-1 points (terminal stages, mute, bedbound, non-interactive)

Descriptors:

Mobility

4 may lurch or have erratic gait, may fall or have near falls, but not daily/multiple times a day

3 falls or bumps into things or has near falls multiple times a day; may wear a helmet, may still walk as primary way to get places, but it scares everyone else! May fall/lurch when standing still

2 uses wheelchair as primary way to get places within residence; moves wheelchair independently (e.g. scoots with the feet)

1 able to sit in a wheelchair, Broda chair, recliner, or other seating arrangement without falling out repeatedly due to chorea, hyperextension, or sliding out. Unable to self-propel a wheelchair

0 unable to sit even in a supported chair, usually because of severe chorea or truncal dyscontrol

Feeding

3 eats already-prepared food using utensils, not just the fingers and hands

2 unable to use utensils properly, but still able to get some food and drink to the mouth (may be messy due to chorea or choking, but self-feeding is the primary means of taking nutrition)

1 most of the food at most meals is conveyed to the mouth by a caregiver, not the patient

0 has a feeding tube in place and uses that as the primary means of taking nutrition

Continence

3   independent and clean

2   independent but not always continent or poor hygiene (may be due to chorea, poor control of volitional movements, or cognitive impairment)

1   incontinent, but participates or tries to participate in performing hygiene

0   incontinent and neither asks for help nor participates actively in hygiene activities

Communication

4   able to interact verbally with people besides family, caregivers; speaks in sentences and phrases that non-intimates can understand

3   still trying to speak, but not very successfully; familial people and those who are aware of the context can get the gist of what is being said, but likely do not understand all the words

2   can communicate simple concepts through single words or short phrases (e.g. "pop" or "I love you" or "%*$#*& you!")

1   unable to say words, but still tries to communicate by sound; grunts or says completely unintelligible noises, may scream to get caregiver's attention or communicate a need

0   mute and appears uninterested in trying to respond orally/verbally in the context of a conversation (e.g., does not grunt, babble, or shriek in response to a question; does not scream when incontinent)

Participation

4   interacts meaningfully with people outside of family/caregivers; participates in household activities

3   limited range of activities or interactions, but still participates actively

2   able to be brought to family or community activities, but does not interact with outsiders, and does not actively engage in the activity (e.g. attends a holiday party but does not sing songs with the family, or is brought to the weekly bingo game but dozes lightly while someone else completes the card)

1   bed-bound or chair-bound, but interacts in a one-on-one situation (e.g. turns when name is called, or hugs back when hugged, or kicks and shoves a caregiver who attempts to bathe or dress him/her)

0   bed-bound and simply stares or remains with eyes closed when addressed or attended to

Superimposed on these measures, which relate to different physical tasks of daily living, are two additional domains: behavioral status, and overall disease stability. Some people with HD have functional restrictions because of severe behavioral disturbance, which can improve if the mood or behavior problems are successfully treated. And it is possible for a person with HD to experience a period of seemingly rapid decline, perhaps in the setting of an acute illness or injury, and then stabilize at a lower functional level for a period of time.

It is important to understand that death due to HD can occur in a person whose total score on the scale in Table 1 is greater than 0; many people with HD, for instance, never use a feeding tube, or have some amount of vocalization even in the terminal stages of their disease.

Management of Late Stage HD

Care Setting

By definition, people in the late stages of HD need 24-hour supervision and assistance with activities of daily living. Behavioral issues dating back to the earlier stages of the disease often lead to burnout among family caregivers. For this reason, and because care partners are often still of an age to have a job (and therefore not available to provide 24-hour care), most people in the late stages of HD are placed outside the home. An occasional person with mild or minimal behavior problems, particularly an older person whose spouse is retired, is able to remain in the home with in-home personal care services or the equivalent from family members. County social service departments, HDSA Center of Excellence social workers, or HDSA Chapter social workers can help a person with HD or family identify day care, respite care, and in-home care services in the community, and to determine whether a person with HD qualifies for financial assistance to pay for them.

For most families, an important hurdle is identifying a long-term care facility that meets the affected individual's needs. Older individuals, and those without behavioral problems, may be appropriately placed in a local facility with ready access to family and friends. Where there are behavior problems, families may find that facilities refuse to take the person with HD; for example, a 40 year old man with impulsive or explosive behavior may not be accepted into a nursing unit where most of the residents are 80 years old and female. Facilities that have units specializing in treating young adults, people with head injuries or psychiatric disturbances may be a better fit for younger people with HD or for those with behavior problems.

Young adults with HD can also sometimes be managed in a group home setting, possibly matched with other people with HD of a similar age, or (depending on the situation), with young adults who have had head injuries or high-functioning developmental delays. Information on long-term care facilities with specific units for residents with HD is available from HDSA, (800) 345-HDSA.

Care Planning for Late Stage HD

People in the late stages of HD have a multifaceted neurological disorder, and typically die from medical complications of the severe neurologic disability. Medical care may best be provided by a team that includes a neurologist or other physician who is knowledgeable about HD and its progression, a psychiatrist or geriatric psychiatrist, familiar with the management of difficult behaviors in the care facility, and an internist who can address the medical complications and co-morbidities. Allied health professionals specializing in nursing, social services, physical therapy, occupational therapy, speech-language pathology, dietetics, psychology, recreational therapy, and music therapy are invaluable resources as the team works to optimize the person's quality of life.

The table on page 104 describes some HD-related symptoms that might necessitate a nursing care plan, and some of the team members who can be involved in the care plan and strategies to improve function or reduce the impact of the symptom. From the nursing perspective, a person with HD will likely need a care plan that includes attention to diet, behavior, communication, safety, hygiene, expert care, management of medical co-morbidities, psychosocial and spiritual care, end-of-life planning, rehabilitation, caregiver support, and risk-sharing with the family.

Movement Disorder

Table 2: Typical movement-related problems seen in late stage HD and the team members who might be called upon to evaluate or assist in the management of the problem as well as typical treatments.

Symptom	Functional result	Team members	Possible management strategy
Chorea	Bruising, abrasions; falling out of chair or bed; entanglement in cords, restraints	MD, OT, nursing, maintenance department	Medications, padding of environment or body, special seats, floor mattress, avoid limb and trunk restraints; remove long cords (such as nurse call lights); frequent monitoring for bruises, skin tears, other injuries
Incoordination of hands, arms	Inability to perform ADLs	OT, nursing	Assistance with ADLs, modified equipment for eating; OT training to optimize function
Gait disturbance	Falls, reduced mobility	PT, OT	Monitor and document falls; pad environment or body, acclimate early to wheelchair; (occasional person can use merrywalker or walker); family communication
Ballistic movements	Falls, limb injury, breaking furniture and toilet	OT, maintenance department	May need Broda or Q foam chair, concrete toilet, other special equipment; low bed or floor mattress
Dystonia	Contractures, impaired oral or perineal hygiene, skin breakdown; inability to eat	Nursing, OT, physician	Botox injections, oral medications, skin care plan, gastrostomy tube

Although people in the late stages of HD may have very severe chorea, severe dystonia may replace chorea. Oral medications do not generally provide satisfying relief of dystonia, but botolinum toxin injections of specific muscles may provide symptomatic relief, easier care, and an improved quality of life.

Volitional movements in the late stages of HD often become few in number, but ballistic in amplitude. This can lead to injury, as people with HD fall or fling themselves into and out of chairs or beds, and onto toilet seats, or crash an arm or leg into a wall, sink, or another person. Medications are generally not helpful, so careful planning of the environment may be necessary. The occupational therapist can assist in identifying heavy-duty furniture or appliances, or creatively padding the chair, bed, walls, furniture corners, or toilet seat. People with severe chorea may need a special nurse alert system, as intentional and non-intentional strangulation on long bedside nurse alert cords has been reported.

Oral-Motor Dysfunction

Table 3: Problems related to oral-motor dysfunction and management strategies.

Symptom	Functional problem	Team members	Possible treatment strategies
Oral motor dysfunction	Dysphagia, drooling, choking, aspiration; weight loss	SLP, nursing, physician, dietitian	Medications/botox for drooling, change food textures, train in safe feeding strategies; increase calorie intake (high calorie supplements); gastrostomy tube; 24-hour access to food
Oral motor dysfunction	Reduced communication skills; mutism	SLP, nursing	Simple word board, computer-based assistive communication device, thoughtful care from staff/family who know person well

Morbidity and death in HD are commonly related to oral-motor dysfunction and resultant dysphagia. Dysphagia can lead to recurrent aspiration pneumonia, weight loss, or "bad behavior" as affected individuals become anxious or frightened around mealtimes, but are unable to express themselves in any other way. It is critical for people who have HD to express an opinion – earlier in the disease course – as to whether they would or would not want a gastrostomy feeding tube placed when they reach that point in their disease (and why or why not). By the time a feeding tube is needed, speech is often so impaired that family and physicians are unable to understand what the individual is trying to say or ask about this somewhat conceptual topic.

The speech-language pathologist (SLP) can perform either a bedside swallow evaluation or a more formal video fluoroscopy study, to assist in determining which textures of foods and liquids are safe, and whether techniques such as the chin tuck, double swallow, or use of straws or "sippy cups" are helpful or not for a particular person. The dietitian can assess caloric needs and recommend specific supplements or foods to use or avoid.

Managing Communication and Dementia-related Problems

Various communication and dementia-based problems can arise in individuals with late stage HD. Managing these problems requires an individualized approach. Two aspects of care are particularly important. The first is to make sure that the person with HD, family, and staff have discussed in advance how the individual would like to be cared for when HD-related dementia has led to an irreversible inability to interact meaningfully, and at what point the person would judge that time to have occurred (some individuals retain social inter-activeness even after they have become mute; others are able to at least make single words or noises to indicate agreement or displeasure). Ideally, the person's wishes regarding care (feeding tubes, etc.) will be documented in an Advance Directive.

The second aspect of care in late stage HD is for the staff to work with the individual or knowledgeable family to document the person's likes and dislikes, and body language, before the person fully loses the ability to interact. In this way, the staff can at least make an educated guess as to the HD person's concern, or how to make him feel better, even if the person no longer interacts verbally. Consistency in staffing can also help to maintain a comforting routine for the individual; it should be expected that changes in staffing may lead to outbursts, or disruptive or resistive behavior.

Dementia

Table 4: Functional problems related to dementia and some management strategies

Symptom	Functional problem	Possible management strategy
Inability to learn	Unable to learn to use adaptive equipment (walker, wheelchair, augmentative communication device, etc)	Introduce equipment early, before the need is critical
Disorientation in time	Day-night confusion	Daytime programming, avoid naps, possible night-time sedative; avoid sedating drugs during the day
Slow processing	Delayed response times	Allow person with HD extra time
Impaired judgment	Dangerous behaviors	Care plans for specific behaviors, know when to call for emergency help, behavioral modification strategies, prn medications
Unawareness/ denial	Dangerous behaviors, confrontational behaviors	Assign staff that person likes/able to handle HD person; care plan for specific behaviors
Apathy/ withdrawal	Lack of interaction, refusal to participate in activities, pressure ulcers, risk of medical complications of inactivity	Rule out depression, consider stimulant drugs, continued encouragement from staff to participate in activities
Communication problems and Dementia	Lack of interaction, mutism	Ensure that Advance Directives are in place before person with HD becomes mute; thoughtful care from staff, family, who have known person

Consultation with a psychologist, psychiatrist, as well as the treating physician, and careful care-planning within the nursing team are critical to successful management of all of these symptoms.

Behavioral-Psychological Symptoms

Table 5: Some behavioral issues and treatment strategies

Symptom	Functional problem	Possible management strategies
Depression	Withdrawal, sadness, suicidality	Medications, counseling, spiritual support, family involvement, suicide risk assessment and documentation
Anxiety	Behavioral over activity, nervousness, substance abuse	Medications, counseling, distracting activities, care plans about cigarette, drug, alcohol use
Paranoia/ Suspiciousness	Resisting care, fights with other residents, overt hallucinations	Change rooms or roommates, behavioral modification, care plans around hygiene, medications (consider IM depot or oral-dissolving preparations)
Irritability	Resistiveness with staff and other residents	Medications, rule out depression, spiritual support, family involvement, environmental strategies
Impulsiveness	Dangerous behaviors, aggressive behaviors	Medications, wanderguard or seat/bed alarm, other environmental strategies
Obsessiveness/ Perseveration	Stickiness (disturbing staff and other residents); smoking	Engage in activities, behavioral modification; smoking cessation using nicotine patches, inhalers, other medications
Explosive/ Aggressive/ violent behavior	Danger to staff and other residents	Care plan for each behavior, identify triggers, know when to call for emergency help, possible prn medications, change roommates or room, engage in other activities
Screaming	Disruptive loud behavior	Evaluate for pain, depression; consider hospice care
Sexually inappropriate behavior	Danger to self or other residents	Careful documentation of behavior, protection of at-risk individuals, environmental changes, pregnancy and STD prevention, rarely medication to reduce libido
Somatic delusions	Non-organic "pain", eating disorder, obsession with bowels, sensation of "skin crawling"	Involvement in distracting activities, psychiatric evaluation, medications
Substance abuse	Undesirable visitors, use of illegal drugs, hoarding pills or alcohol	Involve institution's legal authorities if necessary; enforce rules about visitors, alcohol; consider treatment program

Challenging behaviors are present in some, but by no means all, people with late stage HD. The intensity of behaviors often evolves over time, with an escalation in disturbing behaviors at around the time that a person loses the ability to communicate effectively, and sometimes a decrease in worrisome behaviors as the person becomes more immobile or more demented, and thus less able to generate challenging behaviors.

People in the late stages of HD can respond to and enjoy music and recreational therapies. Communication through music, art, movement, and dance can be particularly therapeutic for the person with HD who is unable to express himself orally. Other people have enjoyed programs in adaptive swimming or horseback riding.

Medical and Psychosocial Issues

Table 6: Some typical medical complications of the late stages of HD

Symptom	Management strategies	Comments
Weight loss	Nutritional supplements, food preferences, gastrostomy tube	Almost universal in late stage HD
Aspiration pneumonia	Medical evaluation, treatment	
Deep-vein thrombosis, pulmonary embolus	Medical evaluation, treatment	Can be a cause of sudden death; related to immobility
Traumatic injury	Emergency referral; avoid situations that lead to injury	Includes broken bones, subdural hematoma, skin tears
Suicidality	Awareness, treatment of depression, emergency referral	Usually occurs earlier in the disease, but can occur in the later stages
Abandonment	Spiritual support, activities, social service to work with the family	The hereditary nature of HD can make visiting an affected parent in the late stages very emotionally challenging
Terminal stages of HD	Hospice care or equivalent	Recognition of terminal stages can be difficult; consider when the person with HD is mute, nonambulatory, losing weight, refusing to eat, or has non-directed screaming

Safety and Autonomy

As the disease progresses, and with certain individuals, it can be very helpful for the care facility to partner with the family in what might be called "risk sharing." Some care decisions are difficult, because of the conflict between the individual's autonomy and the concern for safety or the usual practice, and the potential for risk with either decision.

Table 7: Areas that might require discussion:

Topic	Safety	Autonomy
Aspiration	Use pureed foods or no oral feeds in people with documented severe dysphagia	Preference to eat foods that frequently cause choking; desire not to have a feeding tube
Entanglement	Restraints (bedrails, seatbelts) are not used because of risk of entanglement	Falls out of bed, jumps out of chair, becomes entangled in nurse call light
Food refusal	Suicide precautions, hospitalization, medications, forced feeding	Decision (for example) not to eat, in order to avoid experiencing the terminal stages of HD
Surreptitious use of psychotropic medications	Use of liquid or oral dissolving psychotropic medications in people with severe behavior disturbance who refuse medications and assistance with hygiene	Right to not bathe, to refuse treatments, to engage in behaviors that may present a health hazard to others (e.g. smearing feces or removing clothing in public)
Discontinuing food or tube feedings	Continue tube feedings indefinitely (or discontinue oral feedings in a person who does not want a feeding tube but has severe dysphagia)	Preference by individual or family to continue or discontinue oral or tube feedings
Use of wheelchair	Requiring the use of wheelchair in a person with severe balance problems	Refuses wheelchair, or stands up while belted in the wheelchair, causing worse injury

The Terminal Stages of HD

Barring other health problems, people with HD will eventually reach the terminal stages of their disease. Symptoms that might suggest that a person is reaching the terminal stages include non-ambulatory status, inability or minimal ability to speak or interact, inability to eat, or weight loss.

Because the terminal stages are an expected part of HD, it should be possible to plan ahead for them, to prepare both the family and person with HD for this stage. Because people with HD lose the ability to communicate complex or abstract thoughts in the late stages of the disease, it is important to discuss and make these preparations and care decisions early. People with HD benefit from assigning a trusted individual to make medical and financial decisions on their behalf, when they are no longer able to do so.

Most importantly, though, is the need for people with HD to write Advance Care Directives or assign Medical Power of Attorney to a trusted individual, should they wish to limit any aspect of their health care at any time during their disease course. Many people with HD instruct the medical team not to perform cardio-pulmonary resuscitation or intubation at a certain point in the course of this progressive, fatal neurodegenerative disease. Some want to have a gastrostomy feeding tube placed if they are losing weight or choking, while others prefer not to have such a procedure at this stage of their illness. If the person with HD has not expressed an opinion or preference about a feeding tube, and is not able to communicate by the time the issue arises, then the family is left to make a decision on the person's behalf.

Some people with HD wish to make the unique gift of a brain donation at the time of death. Although the next-of-kin must still provide consent for brain donation at the time of death, it is very helpful to make preliminary arrangements with the Brain Bank or pathologist long before that time, so that the medical care team and family are aware of the individual's desire, and have set in place, in advance, procedures to accomplish the donation efficiently. Contact HDSA for a list of the most current brain banks accepting donations in the U.S. (800-345-4372).

Screaming in Late Stage HD

An observation has been made over the years that a mute and bedbound individual in the late stages of HD who begins to scream has often entered the terminal stages of the disease. Although it is generally impossible to communicate with these individuals, the screaming can be interpreted to mean that the person is experiencing discomfort (either physical or psychological). Of course, *any conclusion* should be supported by examination for treatable sources of discomfort such as broken bones, decubitus ulcers, constipation, bladder infection, etc.

The onset of screaming behavior may indicate the appropriate time to begin hospice care or the equivalent and the family should be notified that the course will be a matter of a few months or less. Transdermal fentanyl or oral long-acting morphine are often the most effective drugs to reduce the screaming and make the person with HD appear more comfortable.

Hospice Care

When it is possible to determine that a person is in the terminal stages of HD and will likely die over the next few days or months, then it is appropriate to consider hospice or palliative care. These care strategies emphasize comfort, freedom from pain, family involvement, and dignity, in place of medical diagnosis and aggressive, invasive, or hospital-based treatment of conditions. The hospice team focuses on the needs of both the affected individual and the family as death approaches. Hospice can be performed in the home, in the hospital, or in a care facility, and most third-party payers pay for hospice services from the benefits that previously or otherwise paid for medical diagnosis and treatment.

110

Unfortunately, there are no written guidelines or even anecdotal descriptions regarding specific treatments to be used or avoided for people with HD as part of palliative or hospice care, so each case must be addressed individually. In general, it is reasonable to consider reduction or discontinuation of medications for prophylaxis of long-term consequences (such as cholesterol medications, osteoporosis treatments, daily aspirin), and vitamins and supplements. Some hospice providers aggressively discontinue all medications (such as blood pressure medications, thyroid medications) except those that are necessary for comfort (which might include diuretics, sleeping pills, and pain pills, among others). It is sometimes unclear how many, and which psychotropic medications, a person with HD who is in hospice should take; these medications may be very important for the psychological comfort of a person who is dying from HD – but the required doses and numbers of medications may be less.

Conversely, abruptly discontinuing medications that a person has taken for a long time can lead to uncomfortable and potentially dangerous rebound symptoms. Thus, caution is recommended as the hospice team attempts to reduce psychotropic medications in a person with HD. The addition of long-acting narcotics has been found to be very helpful for some people with HD who are agitated or who have severe spasticity or dystonia that appears to be painful.

Symptoms that may escalate in the terminal days or weeks include dystonia, drooling, and agitation. Muscle relaxants, anti-cholinergic agents, and anti-anxiety drugs, respectively, may be helpful for these symptoms. Transdermal fentanyl or oral morphine have been found to be the most effective drugs to reduce screaming behavior and make the person appear more comfortable.

Hospice care, especially where there is family involvement, can ease the final days for both the individual and the family.

Summary

Late stage Huntington's Disease occupies a greater portion of the continuum of care than many families or medical professionals may know. Individuals can live for years to a decade or more in the late stage of the disease, needing 24-hour supervision and care.

The importance of planning for late stage Huntington's Disease cannot be overlooked. Physicians and other medical professionals should make an effort to help families prepare, emotionally and financially, for the length of time that their loved one may live in the late stages of the disease.

Delivering long term care for an individual during the late stages of HD can be challenging to both family caregivers and professional caregivers. In addition to assistance with the daily activities of life, individuals in late stage HD may exhibit behavior problems or severe chorea that caregivers will need to work around. Many nursing homes are not equipped to care for persons with late stage HD and it may take time and research to find appropriate placement.

Goals of care remain the same in late stage HD: reduce the burden of symptoms, maximize function and optimize quality of life. It is important that everyone involved in the individual's care remember that dementia in HD is different than in Alzheimer's disease, affecting motor skills and speed of cognitive processing, but not affecting understanding of the meaning of words. Many non-communicative people with late stage HD will still understand what is being said to them and what is going on around them. Older memories are also unaffected and many people in late stage HD are still capable of enjoying reminiscences, photos and scrapbooks.

Because communication in late stage HD becomes so difficult, individuals with the disease should be encouraged to express their feelings about end-of-life care, use of feeding tubes/hydration and other medical issues in an Advance Directive as early as possible.

Case Study: #1

Management of Late Stage HD: Nursing Home Success Story

A 53 year old woman is admitted to the HD unit at the nursing home. She was diagnosed with HD 12 years earlier. She had lived alone in an apartment until three years earlier, when Adult Protective Services became involved because she was dirty, disheveled, and suspected of hoarding. After a psychiatric hospitalization, she was placed in a local nursing home, where she refused medications and terrorized other residents. She was moved to another facility, where she also failed to conform to facility regulations. She was reported to have severe chorea, irritability, unsafe smoking, resisted care and medications, and choked on her food daily. She fell out of bed frequently, and spent her day seat belted into a wheelchair.

After admission to the HD Unit, she was started on an intramuscular anti-psychotic in an attempt to reduce her paranoia and possibly the chorea. Tetrabenazine was considered (as a treatment for chorea), but postponed until her adjustment to the facility was complete. Buproprion and a nicotrol inhaler were used to facilitate smoking cessation, in keeping with institution policy. A speech-language pathologist found that her swallowing problems were due to an impulsive eating style (too large bites, too much liquid without a pause), rather than intolerance of a certain food texture. She was given a cup with a straw, to limit swallow volume, and the staff were instructed to cut her food into small bites. The dietitian assessed her daily caloric needs and recommended high calorie foods as well as nutritional supplements; the woman's food preferences were also identified and made available. She was given a queen-sized bed, and a tilting, heavy, padded recliner (a Broda™ chair) without a seatbelt. Weekly telephone calls were scheduled with her daughter, and the woman was included in music and other creative activities on the unit.

One month later, the woman was no longer smoking, was not falling out of bed, and accepted assistance, with baths and other hygiene from one particular nursing assistant but not others. She had gained 10 pounds, and was a leader of the music group (it turned out that she had been a singer in her high school and church choirs). She was accepting oral medications, and her paranoia had diminished. Her chorea remained severe, and physical therapy was attempting to train her to use a wheelchair independently, as her gait and standing balance were severely impaired.

Case Study: #2

Management of Late Stage HD:
End-of-life and Hospice Care

A 46 year old man affected with HD had lived in a long-term care facility for nine years. The nursing staff reported that he had recently begun to cry out, resist care, and at times, to scream. This was unusual; he was previously "happy-go-lucky," helping other residents and always smiling. He choked frequently during meals, and sometimes threw his plate or hit the aide who was helping him. He was bed-bound, except when he was put in a heavy recliner to watch activities on the nursing unit. His family had stopped calling, frustrated because he was mute and unable to participate in the conversation.

The speech-language pathologist found that he had severe dysphagia for thin liquids but that he could swallow nectar-thick liquids. Nutritional supplements were added, and he was given frequent small meals. He did not have Advance Directives, but lived in a state in which a uniform "Physician Order for Life-Sustaining Treatment" (POLST) document had been developed. The social worker reviewed this document with the man's son, who was his health care agent, and based on this discussion (and views the man had expressed to his family years before), the physician signed an order indicating that the man should not, under any circumstances, have resuscitation attempted, intubation, hospitalization, feeding tube, or IV fluids or antibiotics. After a meeting between the son and a hospice representative, hospice care was initiated.

Cholesterol medication, oxybutinin, and quetiapine were all stopped. A long acting morphine preparation was given, in a low dose, and the man's discomfort appeared to resolve almost completely, so that he was no longer screaming. Family members were encouraged to visit, and with the extra attention of the family and the hospice team, the man briefly rallied. After a few weeks, however, his inter-activeness subsided, and he gradually slipped into a terminal state. With family gathered around, he died five months after hospice care was initiated.

Chapter 9

Clinical Trials and Observational Studies in HD

Vicki Wheelock, M.D.

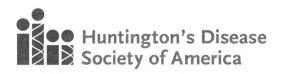
Huntington's Disease
Society of America

Research Participation: Making progress, building hope

When faced with the diagnosis of Huntington's Disease (HD), people with the disease, their families and friends frequently ask the physician what can be done to alleviate symptoms or slow the progression. Providing education about the symptoms and disease course, resources including HDSA Chapters and support groups, scheduling follow-up visits, prescribing medications, therapies, and equipment, and making specialty referrals when indicated are all essential to delivering the best standard of care. Offering people with HD and families the opportunity to participate in clinical research helps to build hope for each person's future as well as for the next generation.

Although the HD gene was discovered in 1993, no effective disease-modifying treatments have yet been discovered. However, clinical research efforts have made significant progress over the ensuing years in developing tools to better define the natural history of HD, including specific motor, cognitive and psychiatric features. A number of clinical trials aimed at developing symptomatic treatments and disease-modifying (neuroprotective) therapies have been completed, and there are currently many active studies in progress. United States government, pharmaceutical industry and private foundation funding for HD clinical research has significantly increased, and new global collaborative efforts are also underway to advance research.

Background and History

Clinical trials include both long-term studies which aim to slow HD progression and short-term studies aimed at symptomatic improvement. Hypotheses for potential HD treatments have been generated by basic scientists determined to find treatments for HD in laboratory models, including robust transgenic mouse models. A large number of basic science researchers have received grants from HDSA. Other organizations have also made significant contributions to HD research. The pioneering Hereditary Disease Foundation (HDF) was founded by Milton Wexler, MD in 1968. The HDF played a key role in recruiting over 100 scientists who worked collaboratively to identify the HD gene by studying pedigrees and blood samples collected from thousands of volunteers in Venezuela, an area with a high prevalence of HD. The National Research Roster for Huntington Disease Patients and Families at Indiana University was founded in 1979. People with HD and their families are invited to volunteer to enroll in the Roster, which acts as a link between people with HD and families and scientists who study HD. The Huntington Study Group was started in 1993 (see below). CHDI is a private, non-profit organization founded in 2005 that seeks to accelerate HD research by funding basic science researchers as well as sponsoring studies developed by the HSG and by the EURO-HD Network.

The Huntington Study Group

The non-profit Huntington Study Group (HSG) was formed in 1993 by a small group of neurologists and researchers led by Dr. Ira Shoulson at the University of Rochester. The mission of the HSG is to carry out cooperative therapeutic research in order to advance knowledge about the natural history and treatment of HD. Guided by an elected Executive Committee, and governed by a constitution and bylaws, the HSG has grown to include over 500 investigators, coordinators and consultants from over 90 sites in the U.S., Canada, Europe, Australia, New Zealand and South America. Since 1993 the HSG has completed 22 clinical trials and observational studies involving over 10,000 participants.

The UHDRS

One of the first HSG goals was to develop a validated rating scale that could be used to assess the clinical features of HD. The Unified Huntington's Disease Rating Scale (UHDRS) was published in 1996. It has six components:

- Motor assessment

- Cognitive assessment

- Behavioral assessment

- Independence scale

- Functional assessment

- Total Functional Capacity (TFC)

The UHDRS has been widely used internationally to establish the natural history of HD and to measure effectiveness of various medications in clinical treatment trials. Longitudinal changes in the Total Functional Capacity subscale of the UHDRS have been studied in order to determine the rate of functional decline in people with HD, critically important as an outcome measure in trials designed to slow HD progression. The motor subscale has been used to measure the effect of interventions on movement-associated features of HD, most notably for chorea. The cognitive subscale has been used to study cognitive performance both before and near the time of diagnosis of HD.

Observational Studies

Observational studies have included a longitudinal UHDRS Natural History Database study with information from more than 8,000 individuals; PHAROS, a pioneering long-term study of people at 50% risk for HD who chose not to know their gene status; PREDICT-HD, a pivotal trial prospectively enrolling people who know their HD gene status and are not yet diagnosed with HD; and more recently COHORT, a study enrolling people who are pre-symptomatic, people diagnosed with HD, their at-risk family members, and control subjects, usually spouses and caregivers who are not at-risk.

The UHDRS Natural History Database has been used to establish a number of important findings, including clinical markers of early disease, rate of functional decline, predictors of nursing home placement, correlates of disability and progression, the contribution of cognitive and psychiatric aspects of HD to functional capacity, correlates of weight loss, depression and stages of HD, critical periods of suicide risk, and predictors of diagnosis.

Milestones in HD observational research studies include the enrollment of 1,001 people who were at 50% risk of inheriting HD and had chosen not to undergo predictive testing in the Prospective Huntington's At-Risk Study (PHAROS), with a baseline publication in 2007. PHAROS findings to date include studies of concerns about health insurance loss, patterns of dietary intake, and attitudes about reproductive choices, with numerous new publications in preparation.

The Predictors of Biologic Markers in HD (PREDICT-HD) study has enrolled more than a thousand individuals who have undergone predictive testing and have the HD gene expansion and are presymptomatic, or who have been found not to have the gene expansion. The goal was to identify changes in markers and behavior before HD is diagnosed. PREDICT-HD succeeded in identifying changes in neuroimaging findings and cognitive test performance years before diagnosis, ushering in the concept of prodromal HD. Additional findings include the identification of motor, psychiatric and functional changes before diagnosis, including a method of identifying presymptomatic gene carriers close to predicted onset of HD using automated brain MRI. PREDICT-HD has also contributed to knowledge about ethical issues related to HD. An additional study, RESPOND-HD, describes the scope of stigmatization and genetic discrimination among participants from the U.S., Canada and Australia enrolled in PHAROS or PREDICT-HD.

PREDICT-HD is focused on the identification of the earliest markers of change in people with the HD gene expansion, with the goal of helping to design future studies of treatments that may delay the onset or slow the progression of HD.

The Cooperative Huntington Observational Research Trial (COHORT) is a study designed to collect longitudinal clinical data and biological samples from individuals with HD and their family members. Funded by CHDI, COHORT has enrolled 3,000 individuals including those with manifest HD, their family members (including those at-risk), and a control group of spouses and caregivers who are not at-risk. Unique options in the study include a family history questionnaire which can identify births, deaths and diagnoses of HD within family members, and the ability to consent to collection and storage of biological samples for future research. The COHORT data set is available to the worldwide HD research community in order to advance the study of HD natural history and biomarkers.

Clinical Trials: Symptomatic Therapies

The TETRA-HD study was designed to determine the safety and efficacy of tetrabenazine for the treatment of chorea. The results, published in 2006, led to the FDA's decision to approve the first drug for HD in the U.S. in 2008. Marketed as Xenazine®, tetrabenazine is now widely prescribed as an anti-chorea drug. A Phase 2 trial of latrepirdine to treat cognitive symptoms in HD (DIMOND) was published in 2009, establishing its safety and tolerability, and there was a suggestion of improvement in cognition. These findings led to a current larger Phase 3 study (HORIZON) of safety and efficacy of latrepirdine co-directed by the HSG and the EURO-HD Network. Additional clinical trials sponsored by the HSG include studies of riluzole, phenylbutyrate, ethyl-EPA, minocycline and ACR-16 (for a description of these studies and their results, please see the HSG website, http://www. huntington-study-group.org/ClinicalResearch/CompletedClinicalTrials/tabid/65/ Default.aspx).

Trials for neuroprotection

Disease-modifying studies to slow HD progression include the study of coenzyme Q10 and remacemide (CARE-HD) published in 2001. While CARE-HD failed to demonstrate a statistically significant reduction of the primary outcome measure, the rate of progression of TFC, there was a suggestion of clinical effectiveness for coenzyme Q10. Subsequent studies at higher doses led to a large NIH-funded trial of high dose coenzyme Q10 in HD, 2CARE, that has enrolled more than 500 people with early stage HD in a 5-year, randomized, placebo-controlled trial.

Another large NIH-funded trial studying the efficacy of high dose creatine to slow HD progression, CREST-E, is also underway. This 3-year, randomized, placebo-controlled clinical trial is for participants with early stage HD. Both 2CARE and CREST-HD are still actively enrolling participants. The first clinical trial for people before the onset of HD was launched in 2009. The PREQUEL study will analyze the safety and tolerability of three different doses of coenzyme Q10 in individuals with the HD gene expansion who are pre-manifest.

Research Horizons

Increasingly, HD clinical research efforts have become global, with organizations including the EURO-HD Network partnering with the HSG on the HORIZON and HART studies. Sponsored by CHDI, ENROLL-HD is an initiative to combine the efforts of the HSG and EURO-HD Network to develop a global observational study, with plans to expand opportunities for participation to sites in Asia and South America. World-wide scientific interest is quite high in developing new HD treatment strategies, include novel therapies designed to modify the huntingtin protein or reduce expression of the huntingtin gene.

Conclusions

Physicians should encourage people with HD and families to consider participation in HD observational studies and clinical trials. Some people and families seek opportunities for research because of their desire to advance progress in finding treatments for HD, while others enjoy the prospect of frequent contact with study personnel and having early access to medications which may be proven effective. Many research volunteers report that participation engenders hope for themselves and for the next generation. However, it is important to recognize that obstacles to research participation also exist for people with HD and families affected by HD, especially given the relatively early age at onset of the disease, as well as the inclusion of people before symptoms appear. Barriers to research participation include travel time and distance to study sites, the need to miss work or childcare duties, concerns about confidentiality, caregiver burden and the challenges of managing HD symptoms day-to-day. The extraordinary number of people who have volunteered to participate in HD research studies attests to the commitment of families to advance HD research. Physicians can play an important role in helping people with HD and families identify opportunities for research participation.

Suggested resources for people with HD and families interested in HD research:
HDSA.org/research/clinical-trials.html
Huntington-Study-Group.org
HDTrials.org
ClinicalTrials.gov

Chapter 10

Appendices

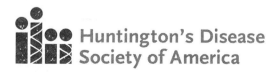
Huntington's Disease
Society of America

Appendix I

Total Functional Capacity Scale (Source: UHDRS)

This scale rates the person's level of independence in five domains: occupation, ability to manage finances, ability to perform domestic chores, ability to perform personal activities of daily living, and setting for level of care. Some clinicians use the TFC score to determine the Shoulson and Fahn rating scale for staging the disease.

Total Functional Capacity Rating Scale[1] (Source: UHDRS[2])		
Domain	**Ability**	**Score**
Occupation	Unable	0
	Marginal work only	1
	Reduced capacity for usual job	2
	Normal	3
Finances	Unable	0
	Major assistance	1
	Slight assistance	2
	Normal	3
Domestic Chores	Unable	0
	Impaired	1
	Normal	2
Activities of Daily Living	Total care	0
	Gross tasks only	1
	Minimal impairment	2
	Normal	3
Care level	Full-time nursing care	0
	Home for chronic care	1
	Home	2
TOTAL	Range 0 - 13	

Shoulson and Fahn Staging Scale[1]

TFC Total Score	Stage
11 - 13	I
7 - 10	II
3 - 6	III
1 - 2	IV
0	V

1   Shoulson I, Kurlan R, Rubin AJ et al. Assessment of functional capacity in neurodegenerative movement disorders: Huntington's disease as a prototype, in Munsat TL (ed): Quantification of Neurological Deficit. Boston: Butterworth, 1989, pp 271-283.

2   The Huntington Study Group. Unified Huntington's Disease Rating Scale: reliability and consistency. Mov Disord 1996; 11:136-142.

UHDRS Motor Assessment Chorea Scale

Assessing chorea, before and after treatment with a medication, is often done using the Unified Huntington's Disease Rating Scale (UHDRS), a research tool which has been developed by the Huntington Study Group (HSG) to provide a uniform assessment of the clinical features and course of HD. The UHDRS has undergone extensive reliability and validity testing and has been used as a major outcome measure by the HSG in controlled clinical trials. Information on obtaining the entire UHDRS may be found on the HSG website, www.huntington-study-group.org, by clicking on the Resources tab.

The UHDRS includes a subscale for assessing motor disorders. Chorea is rated in one of seven body regions. The total chorea score is the sum of the scores for each body region, and can range from 0 – 28.

Unified Huntington's Disease Rating Scale Motor Assessment Chorea Scale		
Body Region	**Severity**	
Face	0	Absent
Bucco-oral-lingual	1	Slight/intermittent
Trunk	2	Mild/common or moderate/intermittent
Right upper extremity	3	Moderate/common
Left upper extremity	4	Marked/prolonged
Right lower extremity	Total score: Sum of scores for each body region Range = 0 - 28	
Left lower extremity		

Appendix II

Chapter Notes

Since there is currently only one FDA approved treatment for a symptom of Huntington's Disease, all medications and treatments cited in this guide are used "off label" by the authors.

Chapter 1: Overview and Principles of Treatment

A Systematic Review of the Treatment Studies in Huntington's Disease since 1990
Peter Bonelli and Peter Hofman
University Clinic of Psychiatry, Graz Medical University, Auenbruggerplatz 31, A-8036 Graz, Austria
Expert Opin.Pharmacother.(2007) 8(2): 141-153

Chapter 3: Team Care for Huntington's Disease

EHDN Guidelines for Physiotherapists/Physical Therapy
This evidence-based document aims to provide a uniform standard of care in the area of physical therapy for people with HD. The recommendations that are made in the document are based on a systematic approach to gathering and reviewing currently available literature as well as gathering expert consensus from within the European HD Network.

Date of publication of first edition: February 2010. To access it, go to www.euro-HD.net and click on "Working Groups" and then "physiotherapy" or email info@euro-hd.net.

Chapter 5: The Cognitive Disorder

There have been several published articles over the past 24 months that report outcomes of the PREDICT-HD study. Please conduct an internet search for a complete list of published articles as they relate to the earliest symptoms of HD.

Chapter 7: Juvenile Onset HD

Peter S. Harper, 1996. Huntington's Disease, 2nd Edition, WB Saunders: London

Appendix III

Resource Directory

Guide to HDSA's Centers of Excellence

HDSA Centers of Excellence serve as the cornerstone of HDSA's commitment to care. These 21 facilities provide a vast array of medical and social services to HD families nationwide and work in collaboration with HDSA Chapters, Affiliates, regions and support groups to form a seamless national network of resources and referrals for those affected by HD and their families.

HDSA Centers of Excellence also offer family members the opportunity to be part of the search for effective treatments and a cure through clinical trials. As research advances, there will be a greater need for individuals who want to be a part of finding the answers. Interesting clinical and observational trials are being conducted at every HDSA Center of Excellence. To find out more about the clinical trials available in your area, please visit the HDSA National website, www.hdsa.org, Huntington Study Group web site at www.huntington-study-group.org, or call your closest HDSA Center of Excellence.

Please note that information does change from time to time. Please visit the HDSA web site for the most current contact information (click on "Living with Huntington's Disease"/"Centers of Excellence").

NEW ENGLAND REGION

New England HDSA Center of Excellence
Charlestown, MA

GREATER NEW YORK REGION

HDSA Center of Excellence at University of Rochester
Rochester, NY

**HDSA Center of Excellence at Columbia Health Sciences/
NYS Psychiatric Institute**
New York, NY

**George C. Powell HDSA Center of Excellence at
North Shore University Hospital**
Manhasset, NY

MID-ATLANTIC REGION

HDSA Center of Excellence at Johns Hopkins University
Baltimore, MD

HDSA Center of Excellence at University of Virginia Health System
Charlottesville, VA

SOUTHEAST REGION

HDSA Center of Excellence at Emory University
Atlanta, GA

HDSA Center of Excellence at University of South Florida
Tampa, FL

HDSA Center of Excellence at University of Alabama
Birmingham, AL

GREAT LAKES REGION

HDSA Center of Excellence at the Ohio State University
Columbus, OH

HDSA Center of Excellence at Washington University School of Medicine
St. Louis, MO

HDSA Center of Excellence at Indiana University
Indianapolis, IN

HDSA Center of Excellence at Rush University Medical Center
Chicago, IL

SOUTH CENTRAL REGION

HDSA Center of Excellence at Baylor College of Medicine
Houston, TX

HDSA Center of Excellence at the Colorado Neurological Institute
Englewood, CO

UPPER MIDWEST REGION

HDSA Center of Excellence at Hennepin County Medical Center
Minneapolis, MN

HDSA Center of Excellence at University of Iowa Hospitals and Clinics
Iowa City, IA

NORTHWEST REGION

HDSA Center of Excellence at University of Washington
Seattle, WA

PACIFIC SOUTHWEST ERGION

HDSA Center of Excellence at University of California
Davis Medical Center
Sacramento, CA

HDSA Center of Excellence at University of California
Los Angeles, CA

HDSA Center of Excellence at University of California
San Diego, CA

HDSA Social Workers

HDSA provides social services through its HDSA Centers of Excellence program and its Chapters and Affiliates. To find a social worker in your area, please consult the list below. However, because information changes frequently, we suggest that you visit the HDSA national web site at www.hdsa.org and click on "Living with HD" and then "social workers."

NEW ENGLAND REGION

MASSACHUSETTS

New England HDSA Center of Excellence
Charlestown, MA

HDSA New England Regional Office

GREATER NEW YORK REGION

NEW YORK

**HDSA Center of Excellence at Columbia Health Sciences/
New York State Psychiatric Institute**
New York, NY

**George C. Powell HDSA Center of Excellence at
North Shore University Hospital**
Great Neck, NY

HDSA Center of Excellence at University of Rochester
Rochester, NY

MID-ATLANTIC REGION

DISTRICT of COLUMBIA

HDSA Washington Metro Chapter
Fairfax, VA

DELAWARE

HDSA Delaware Valley Chapter
Plymouth, PA

MARYLAND

**HDSA Center of Excellence at Johns Hopkins
Johns Hopkins Hospital**
Baltimore, MD

PENNSYLVANIA

HDSA Delaware Valley Chapter
Plymouth, PA

HDSA Western Pennsylvania Chapter
Pittsburgh, PA

VIRGINIA

HDSA Center of Excellence at University of Virginia
Charlottesville, VA

SOUTHEAST REGION

ALABAMA

HDSA Center of Excellence at University of Alabama
Birmingham, AL

FLORIDA

HDSA Center of Excellence at the University of South Florida
Tampa, FL

GEORGIA

HDSA Center of Excellence at Emory University School of Medicine
Atlanta, GA

GREAT LAKES REGION

ILLINOIS

HDSA Center of Excellence at Rush University Medical Center
Chicago, IL

INDIANA

HDSA Center of Excellence at Indiana University School of Medicine
Indianapolis, IN

HDSA Indiana Chapter
Indianapolis, IN

KENTUCKY

HDSA Kentucky Chapter
Louisville, KY

MICHIGAN

HDSA Michigan Chapter
Dimondale, MI

MISSOURI

HDSA Center of Excellence at Washington University School of Medicine
St. Louis, MO

OHIO

HDSA Center of Excellence at Ohio State University
Columbus, OH

HDSA Ohio Valley Chapter
Cincinnati, OH

HDSA Northeast Ohio Chapter
Twinsburg, OH

WISCONSIN

HDSA Wisconsin Chapter
Wauwatosa, WI

UPPER MIDWEST REGION

IOWA

HDSA Center of Excellence at University of Iowa Hospitals and Clinics
Iowa City, IA

MINNESOTA

Minnesota Chapter
Fridley, MN

HDSA Center of Excellence at Hennepin County Medical Center
Minneapolis, MN

NORTH DAKOTA

HDSA Northern Plains Affiliate
Grand Forks, ND

SOUTH DAKOTA

HDSA Sioux Valley Chapter
Sioux Falls, SD

SOUTH CENTRAL REGION

COLORADO

HDSA Center of Excellence at the Colorado Neurological Institute
Engelwood, CO

HDSA Rocky Mountain Chapter
Wheat Ridge, CO

TEXAS

HDSA Center of Excellence at Baylor College of Medicine
Houston, TX

HDSA Texas Chapter
Dallas, TX

NORTHWEST REGION

WASHINGTON

HDSA Center of Excellence at University of Washington
Seattle, WA

HDSA Northwest Chapter
Seattle, WA

PACIFIC SOUTHWEST REGION

ARIZONA

HDSA Arizona Affiliate
Glendale, AZ

CALIFORNIA

HDSA Center of Excellence at University of California, Davis Medical Center
Sacramento, CA

HDSA Center of Excellence at University of California
San Diego, CA

HDSA Center of Excellence at UCLA
Los Angeles, CA

HDSA CHAPTERS

HDSA has 8 regional development offices staffed with professionals who work with HDSA Chapters and Affiliates to fulfill the Society's mission to improve the lives of people living with Huntington's Disease.

Information changes constantly. Please visit the HDSA web site at www.hdsa.org and click on "Find HDSA in Your Community" for an up to date listing of contact information for each of the regions noted below.

NEW ENGLAND REGION (ME, NH, VT, CT, MA, RI)

Maine Affiliate

New Hampshire Affiliate

Massachusetts Chapter

Connecticut Affiliate

Rhode Island Affiliate

GREATER NEW YORK REGION (NY, NJ)

Upstate New York Chapter

Greater New York Chapter

New Jersey Chapter

MID-ATLANTIC REGION (DE, MD, DC, PA, WVA, VA)

Delaware Chapter

Washington Metro Chapter

Delaware Valley Chapter

Western Pennsylvania Chapter

SOUTHEAST REGION (NC, SC, GA, FL, TN, AL)

North Carolina Chapter

Georgia Chapter

South Florida Chapter

Central Florida Affiliate

North Florida Affiliate

GREAT LAKES REGION (IL, IN, KY, MI, MO, OH, WI)

Illinois Chapter

Indiana Chapter

Kentucky Chapter

Michigan Chapter

St. Louis Chapter

Northeast Ohio Chapter

Ohio Valley Chapter

Central Ohio Chapter

Wisconsin Chapter

UPPER MIDWEST REGION (MN, IA, NB, ND, SD)

Minnesota Chapter

Iowa Chapter

Sioux Valley Chapter

Northern Plains Affiliate

SOUTH CENTRAL REGION (AR, CO, LA, MS, NM, OK, TX, KS)

Rocky Mountain Chapter

Oklahoma Chapter

Texas Affiliate

NORTHWEST REGION (ID, MT, OR, WY, WA)

Northwest Chapter

PACIFIC SOUTHWEST REGION (AZ, UT, NV, CA)

Arizona Affiliate

Northern California Chapter

Orange County Chapter

Los Angeles Chapter

San Diego Chapter

NOTES

NOTES

NOTES

NOTES